BOOMER YOGA

Energizing the Years Ahead for Men & Women

BERYL BENDER BIRCH

Author of the bestselling *Power Yoga*

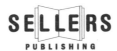

SELLERS
PUBLISHING

Published by Sellers Publishing, Inc.
Copyright © 2009 Beryl Birch Bender
All rights reserved

161 John Roberts Road, South Portland, Maine 04106
For ordering information:
(800) 625-3386 toll free
(207) 772-6814 fax
Visit our Web site: www.sellerspublishing.com
E-mail: rsp@rsvp.com

Edited by: Mark Chimsky-Lustig
Book design: Heather Zschock
Production: Charlotte Smith
Front cover photograph, spine, and glossary photographs: © 2009 François Gagné
www.francoisgagne.com
Back cover author photograph: © 2009 Laura Berland
All other photography: © 2009 Hollis O. Haywood
and Bernard Meyers Photography
www.meyersphoto.com

ISBN: 13: 978-1-4162-0542-5
Library of Congress Control Number: 2008908830

10 9 8 7 6 5 4 3 2 1

Printed in the United States of America.

The information in this book is not meant to replace the guidance
or treatment of your health care providers. Always consult your physician
about matters regarding your personal health, especially before
embarking on an exercise routine.

CONTENTS BOOMER YOGA

Introduction BOOMER YOGA

The whole idea for *Boomer Yoga* started when I realized that I couldn't exactly do what I used to do in terms of physical activity. *My body is changing. Oh my God.* That was one hell of a realization. I mean, I wasn't exactly geriatric but there were subtle alterations. And it wasn't about discovering a gray hair or a wrinkle. Those things don't seem to bother me. Since my primary physical activity was a pretty athletic form of the yoga *asanas* (the practice of the yoga postures) that I had been doing since 1980 and that had inspired my first book, *Power Yoga*, it was in my yoga practice that I first began to notice changes to my body. Those subtle changes had probably been going on for some time. And now they had become a little less subtle.

In the past, I resisted change like mad and went ballistic when unfortunate things happened. I found that that really didn't get me too far. After years of practicing being with what is, as yoga directs us to do, I sat down, face to face, with change. One day, just after coming out of rest at the end of my yoga practice, I sat up laughing. My right hip was really bothering me and restricting my range of motion. I thought to myself, *Oh boy, I'll have to start teaching boomer yoga, a practice for all of us whose bodies are changing.* Boom, there ya go — that's how it happens, a bolt from the blue — "boomer yoga." I'm a couple of years ahead of the first boomers, but as I sat there still chuckling to myself, it occurred to me that if this was happening to me, there were a whole bunch of folks out there, part of the most successful and prosperous generation ever, who were going to be coming up on some big changes. And all their money and "stuff," their apparent security, were not going to bring them the satisfaction they had hoped it would. That satisfaction would only come from knowing who they are, and what really matters in their lives. And ultimately, that's what yoga teaches.

So this book is for all of us — the baby boomers — born between 1946 and 1964. Who are we? Well, we are a powerful group, we do know that much because we sure get a lot of attention from a lot of different venues. We know that we aren't our parent's generation. We aren't geriatric, at least not yet. We are healthier, we are living longer, and we are doing stuff our parents never dreamed of. We have spent a lot of time working on success. We have lots of nice things. We have beautiful homes. We've weathered tough times and survived. Our kids are growing or grown and having kids of their own. And now we are looking around thinking, *Okay, I've done this "success" thing. I'm comfortable, I've prospered, I've accumulated some sense of "security," but I'm not quite all that satisfied. There is something gnawing away at me, a restlessness, a subterranean yearning to know the deeper meaning of life.* There is a movement we can feel, a perceptible but welcome shift.

For all of you who are moving into the middle of life and noticing change — maybe for the first time, maybe for awhile now, or maybe not yet — here is an extraordinary, simple, ancient methodology that will help you to know your True Self. This is not a one-size-fits-all-yoga-class. This is a means for evolution, your own evolution. Where it takes you is where it takes you. It will be different for everyone who climbs on board. Whether you have been doing an *asana* yoga practice for years and years or have always wanted to try yoga, this can point you in the right direction easily and gently. Whether you want to develop the strongest *asana* practice you can or tone down a blazing training routine you've been doing for years, boomer yoga can help you to turn up the heat or dial it down. The practice will slowly lead you through each of the eight limbs of classical yoga and help you move from the postures (*asana*) to energy control (*pranayama*) to concentration (*dharana*) and meditation (*dhyana*). So, whether you're starting a regular meditation practice for the first time or you've been practicing meditation for a long time, here is a tool, a method to follow that will easily bring you greater health, stability, balance, and peace of mind.

But the biggest thing I hope you will learn from *Boomer Yoga* is that *asana* is the equivalent of kindergarten in yoga. It is important to do for life, for health and fitness, but it is still only a small part of what is meant by yoga. *Asana* is only meant to be an aid to preparing us for the deeper work of yoga, specifically meditation. Can *asana* keep us healthy, agile and pliable, and more resistant to injury in our sports activities and everyday life? No question. And that is certainly why we get started in yoga and an important reason we continue. But it's still only a gateway to a vast unlimited awareness of our own boundlessness. That is the experience of yoga. The *Boomer Yoga* routine takes only 40 minutes, but the true practice of it, of learning to be fully present, happens 24/7.

Beryl Bender Birch
East Hampton, New York
December, 2008

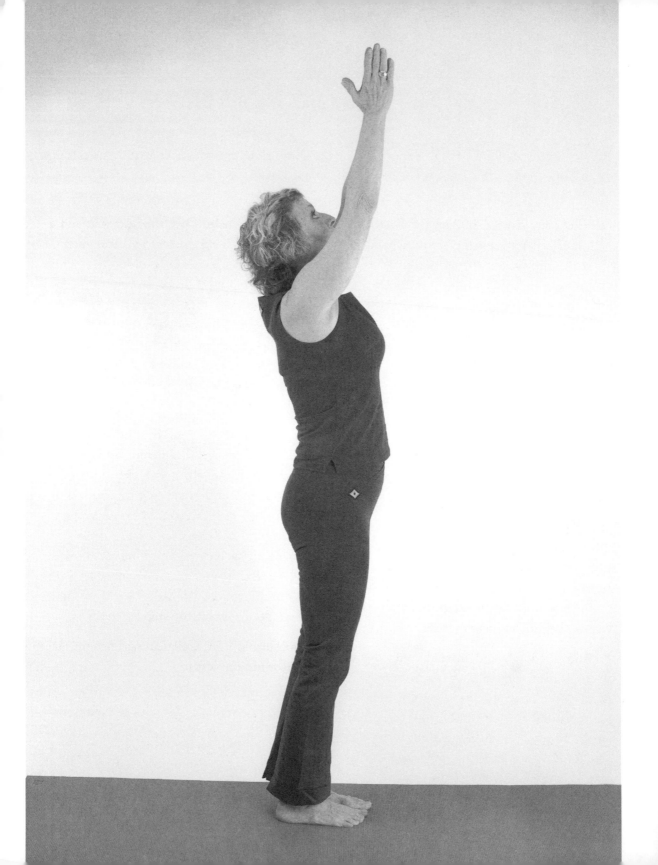

Chapter 1   SHIFT HAPPENS

Taking Charge of Change

One February day in 2002 on the East End of Long Island, when there was a break in the dreary gray winter cold, the sun came out and the temperature went up into the high forties. I went out for a very easy ride on my mountain bike with a friend. I'm not really a mountain biker, despite having a mountain bike which I pedal around on the roads, so I was being extremely conscious of not overdoing it on the meandering trails of East Hampton. But about a week later, I noticed this little tweak in my right groin. I supposed I'd just strained my *psoas* (a hip flexor) muscle from doing a little too much on the ride. And as always, with any little injury I'd ever had in the past twenty-two years, whether from running, biking, swimming, dog sledding, or just doing stuff, I figured that a few weeks of regular practice of the yoga *asanas*, or "postures," would fix the problem. But after a few weeks, the problem wasn't fixed.

I avoided biking, and instead, walked and swam in the Bay during that summer. I tried more *asana*, less *asana*, and finally, no *asana* but the pull persisted. This was getting aggravating. I'd never experienced not being able to "fix" something that was amiss in my body. Grrrrr. By the fall, I conceded I needed

some outside help. Over the next year and a half I went to a chiropractor, an acupuncturist, a massage therapist, and a body tuner — numerous times — and still there was no improvement. In fact, the pain got worse. Every time I *adducted*, or brought my leg in toward the other one (as in getting in and out of a car and as in just about everything else I did) there was a sharp stabbing sort of pain in my groin. Yikes.

Two years later, almost to the day, in February of 2004, I decided I needed serious medical diagnosis and went to see Dr. Lisa Callahan, an orthopedist and medical director of the Women's Sports Medical Center at the Hospital for Special Surgery in New York City. I'd never been to an orthopedist, didn't have medical insurance, and didn't really ever see doctors, except for my gynecologist once a year. So this was a big step for me.

"It's your hip," Dr. Callahan said briskly, as I walked into the office.

"I beg your pardon?" I said, looking around the office to see who she might be talking to.

She came highly recommended by a friend who works at Weill Cornell Medical College at New York Presbyterian and had suggested that I check out the Women's Sports Medicine Center. I must have looked puzzled. Had she seen my X-rays already? I wondered.

"Your hip — it's your hip," she repeated.

"It's not my hip. The pain is here, in the *psoas* muscle," I explained patiently, hoping to be helpful. I pointed to my groin. "Every time I flex my hips (bend over) or *adduct,* I get a sharp, grabbing pain in my groin."

"Yeah, I understand, but it's not your *psoas* muscle," she continued. "It's your hip."

"Did you look at the X-rays?"

"I don't need to look at the X-rays — I can tell by the way you are walking."

"What's wrong with the way I'm walking?"

"Did you know you're limping?" she asked.

"I'm not limping."

"You *are* limping a bit," she replied.

"How do you know?"

"I just watched you walk into this office."

At that point, a technician walked into her office with my X-rays. She put them up on the light board and as the photons illuminated my bones, we looked them over. "Hmmmm," she groaned. "Oooooh, you see this, here?" There was a pretty substantial bone spur off the front, lower portion of the head of the femur, or thigh bone, where it fits into the hip joint. That bone spur is what was causing the problem. It was catching on one of the hip flexor muscles, during flexion or adduc-

tion, and causing that sharp pain I'd been feeling for the past two years. The hip joint was a bit worn looking. "You have osteoarthritis," she explained. "It's in both hips, but its worse in your right hip. You'll probably need a hip replacement in ten years."

Excuse me? I was stunned. She had to be mistaken. I'm Beryl Bender Birch, I don't do "hip replacements," much less osteoarthritis. What was she talking about? How can I have a bone spur? Bone spurs happen when there is some misalignment. I'm a yogi. How can I possibly be misaligned? I just gazed dully at the X-rays. I don't remember the rest. I was polite, as I usually am in these circumstances. But I immediately zoned out. I wasn't really there. She gave me a prescription for something. I don't know what. I just remember walking back to my car, parked in some gloomy underground lot on the Upper East Side of Manhattan, and then driving one hundred miles east to the end of Long Island and home. I just couldn't get my brain around what was happening here.

I was in shock. *How could this be? She had to be kidding.* Hip replacement? I felt like I'd been hit by a truck. I had been practicing yoga since 1971 and teaching it for thirty years. I'd worked with thousands upon thousands of athletes. I'd helped hundreds of runners, bikers, climbers, skiers, and others heal injuries and return to full capacity using a strong physical yoga practice called *astanga* and its modifications (what I called "power yoga") as a form of physical and mental therapy. My book, *Power Yoga*, had sold more than 200,000 copies and had started tons of people on the yoga path to balance and well-being. Personally, I had always believed there was nothing that could not be fixed with regular yoga practice and a little supportive body work.

I eat well, very well. I don't eat saturated fats. I've never had margarine, and I don't eat Wonder bread, soda, canned anything (except tomatoes in the winter for soup), or luncheon meat. I haven't had a piece of bacon or a hot dog since 1958. I avoid high glycemic foods. I haven't eaten anything processed since the '50s, when Velveeta cheese was "invented" and became the saving grace of every house-wife raising children (including my mother) and the magic ingredient of macaroni and cheese. Since I was a child, I've been eating veggies like kohlrabi, kale, and Swiss chard and grains like millet and quinoa that, until recently, most people had never heard of. I've been supporting local organic farming for thirty-five years. I practice yoga. I don't get injured and if I do, I get better by doing yoga. I help other people deal with their injuries. I can see misalignments in *other* people before they even tell me what's wrong with them. I don't get osteoarthritis! And I don't get bone spurs.

As you can tell, I was in denial. It's what generally happens in these cases. It's often the first phase of our response to bad news. But it is often hard to recognize. You don't know if you are in denial or just trying to think positively. So I didn't really deliberate the diagnosis, except when I was bending over, my groin seized up and I yelped and jumped. The dust settled. I didn't have health insur-ance. I hadn't had health insurance since 1974 or '75, when I was still in the Screen Actors Guild. I didn't get sick and I didn't do hip replacements. Somebody told me that a hip replacement cost about the same as a brand new Cadillac. I moved out of denial. I was now depressed.

What was I going to do? Well, I couldn't bend over, so most of my yoga practice was basically not doable. The Sun Salutations were painful for me — especially stepping forward into a lunge position. Ummmm, not great. The hip hurt. I took to calling the injury "my hip." It kind of loomed large in my mind, especially when I tried to do some of the Standing Postures in yoga, where you have to bend over, like Triangle Posture and Extended Side Angle — oooohhh, not so good. People asked how I was and I told them I had osteoarthritis *and* a bone spur. "It's my hip." People were polite. But I felt like I'd failed somehow. I was supposed to be this paragon of wellness. I was a yoga teacher and now I could hardly even practice *asana* myself!

How could this have happened? One of the things Dr. Callahan did happen to ask me while I was in her office was if I had ever been in an auto accident. Well, yes, I recalled, a little one. Sometime in the mid-'80s, when my husband Thom and I had been living in a small cottage on an estate in New Canaan, Connecticut. We had been out on a rainy day, teaching yoga at the Stamford Y and while driving home on wet roads, a car in front of us delivering Meals on Wheels came to an abrupt halt. I was a passenger, no seat belt, and all of a sudden, going about 25 mph, we hit the brakes and skidded into the back of the stopped car. I was thrown forward. My knee, which was higher than my hip, as knees tend to be when you're sitting in a car, hit the dash, pushing my right hip back and down. And as I spoke with Dr. Callahan, there it was — the aha moment — the source of the osteoarthritis and bone spur. That revelation was so beneficial to have, as it helped me to become more tolerant of misalignment and imperfection — especially my own! Over the years, I have pretty much managed to keep the osteoarthritis at bay through careful diet and nutritional awareness. The hip replacement hasn't happened yet, and through a great nutritional protocol and yoga practice, I'm not in pain, still moving, and very grateful.

EXCHANGING ATOMS

Sitting in the front seat of the front car of the boomer generation train, this is what I've figured out about getting older. Our bodies, our minds, our interests, our abilities, all are changing. It is undeniable. The body *is* really slowing down — whether it begins to happen at forty-five or at sixty-five, it happens. Our perspective and passions change. The change is irrefutable and the longer we resist noticing, the more out of touch we are with our whole process of personal evolution. We are *supposed* to change, everything in the world of form changes — things come into existence

and things go out of existence and we will all pass along. It's not depressing. It's life. It can be difficult or easy. Only one thing determines which it will be — our own resistance or compliance.

The choice happens every second — we can join in, or we put up our hands and push against the flow. What I've found is that if you resist, you miss out on the whole reality of life. If you comply, you join in the flow, and you can even direct the rudder as to which direction you'd like to go. By not resisting I don't mean you just accept any injustice, any abuse, or any illegal act that comes your way. I am *not* saying that there aren't some things in life that will make us unhappy or uncomfortable — and given the current state of our global condition, there certainly are plenty. But until you get present with them, you can't do anything about them. Accepting what is, simply because it *is*, and then doing the work for transformation, moment by moment, day by day, is the way of true yoga. But the first step is to be present all the while with each moment, as it is.

There is a Sanskrit word, *maya*, which is used often in the Eastern wisdom traditions that generally means "illusion." But a more technical definition, from a quantum physics point of view, would be something that gives the appearance of "non-change" but in actuality is changing very rapidly. That's us and our world. We think we are solid and quite permanent — especially when we are younger. But in reality (and I mean this literally, not figuratively) we are not the same person physically that we were when we began reading this chapter five minutes ago. We think we have these very well-defined, permanent edges, solid boundaries that separate us from everything else out there. But our edges are anything but well-defined and the solid boundaries are as elusive and empty as galactic space.

Our body is actually a *field* of energy, not a solid clump of matter, and if we could view it from the perspective of a quantum physicist, it would look like a huge empty void with a few specks and fragments and squiggly, random electrical discharges. This field of energy we call *home*, our body, is in dynamic exchange with the rest of the Universe, which is also a field of energy — only a huge, infinite field. The rock-solid being that we think we are is actually in the process of exchanging atoms — every last one of them — with everything around itself. As Deepak Chopra writes in his book *Buddha*, the Buddha said, "Look at the forest. We walk through it every day and believe it to be the same forest. But not a single leaf is the same as yesterday. Every particle of soil, every plant and animal, is constantly changing. You cannot be enlightened as the separate person you see yourself to be because that person has already disappeared, along with everything else from yesterday."

Dr. Chopra gives the example of breathing to illustrate this process of exchange. He says that every time we breathe in we take in 10 to the 22nd power number of atoms, and every time we breathe out we do the same. We breathe in millions upon millions of atoms from all around us which become parts of our liver, our heart, our brain cells, etc. And when we breathe out we give off atoms that were parts of our liver and heart and skin cells, etc. As Dr. Chopra says, "We make a new liver every six weeks." That means that every single atom in your liver tissue is exchanged with others that you have taken in through breathing and eating, and the ones you are getting rid of are off-loaded through elimination and breathing. And this happens every six weeks! (However, it's not the same thing as a liver transplant. The intelligence and information contained in the "field" of the cells and the DNA is thought, at present, to stay the same. So the existing condition of the liver will continue even with the arrival of new atoms. But at some point in the future, who knows, maybe we could energetically create a new liver!) It really is an amazing concept to contemplate. Last month, the neurons in your brain might have been in a tree or in your boss's colon. Happy thought, eh? But it's true.

According to Dr. Chopra, we all have atoms in our bodies that once were in the body of Christ or Buddha — or Genghis Khan for that matter. Quite literally, we are part of a cosmic body that is constantly in exchange with its own Self. There are no real edges to us, no boundaries — just swirling fluctuations of energy. I often sit, quietly, sometimes before meditation, and see if I can visualize these atoms bursting out of my field of energy into the Universe — becoming available to whatever happens to drift by.

PUSHING AGAINST WHAT IS

When facing huge, obvious, in-your-face change, I've found that we have two basic options: we either "get with the program" and accept the change, celebrate it even, or we get stuck in the mud of resistance and miss out on the only reality there is — right here, right now. If you are stuck in the mud, the first thing you need to acknowledge is, "Yes, here I am, stuck in the mud." From there the right action can develop. But if the first reaction is thrashing and crashing about — no, no, no, this can't be happening — then you impale yourself in the mire and could drown in the cacophony you've created. And there is generally plenty of cacophony going on that we aren't crazy about: our teenage daughter just wrecked the car, someone we love has been diagnosed with cancer, the dog ran away, the computer crashed, the boss freaked out, or the power has been out for a week. It's funny — when you resist what *is* by being unhappy with whatever is going on at the moment, you completely lose touch with life.

Good or bad, gain or loss, the only way you can do anything about anything going on is — first of all — you've got to be *there*!!! It may not be so comfortable to be *there*. More than likely you will completely get caught up in the swirlings of the mind, thinking how it should be different, and that struggle to resist will take you anywhere but *there*. "This is awful. How could this happen? What was she thinking? What will I do? What is wrong with him?" And so the mind buzzes. The energy output is phenomenal. We fight like mad to avoid being caged in that unpleasant, painful moment.

The Yoga Sutra, the ancient text on yoga, tells us that the avoidance of pain, or *dvesa*, is a form of "ignorance," or *avidya*. What? It's ignorant to avoid pain? That's crazy. Why would yoga counsel that philosophy? I don't want pain in my life, is what most of us think and feel. Certainly, trying to avoid pain has to be a good thing. After all, what about our survival? If we experience something that damn near kills us, we will probably be cautious about repeating that encounter. How could that be "ignorance"?

Well, *The Yoga Sutra* is looking at it in a slightly less basic way. If we are ruled or governed to any degree by an aversion to things we don't like or are "painful," it limits our life experience. No problem, you might think, I don't mind limiting my life experience if it is pain-free. But isn't that really cheating our life? Isn't it being disrespectful to this incredible life we have been given, this amazing opportunity to evolve and grow and experience life in all its fullness, (and yes, even do yoga) if we set conditions on what we will allow into our life experience? And whoa, hold the phone! What we haven't even mentioned yet are all the good things that come about as a result of our "painful" experiences. Isn't it true that our moments of greatest insight and most exponential growth come as a result of our "dark nights of the soul"? Oh drat, I guess that is true! Really, we should embrace discomfort. Unfortunately, we rarely do until *after* the pain passes — only then can we see the light.

Yoga will try to teach us to be less *discomfortable* with discomfort — a handy skill to acquire. The fact that we expect our life to be pain-free, or all about pleasure and gain and praise, is what gives birth to the "ignorance" part!! Painful things happen and they are painful for us because in many cases they represent losing something or someone. Yoga tells us that because we don't really understand that *everything* in this world is *impermanent* and it will all return to an "unmanifest" state, then we are being "ignorant" of the true nature of things. We are not seeing the world around us clearly but through a filter created by our own likes and dislikes, which will only lead to more pain and suffering.

Our experiences, good or bad, sort of "layer" into our lives, but they don't just gather on the horizon and sit there piling up. They build on one another in a more holographic way. They move us forward, and also "up and out," in a kind of ascending spiral, expanding our awareness and range of possibility. So we won't ever be in exactly the *same* place or *same* situation again — it's impossible. We have additional experiences, karmas, beliefs, and memories that will influence the moment. So we can't really experience the same pain in the same way — ever.

But as we grow and get older, we begin to understand some of this and recognize how life works. That's why this book is written, not for teenagers, not for twentysomethings, but for you, adults who have been through a good part of life and are starting to "get" some of the things we have been talking about. You are noticing the change and expansion and evolution in your lives. You are a little more deeply curious about what it is you are doing here in the first place. You want to know just who you really are.

Of course, we recognize that our bodies have been changing since the day we were born, and perhaps now we realize that we are changing faster than we can even imagine. But we are also noticing a different type of change — injuries that take longer to heal, bodies that are a bit stiffer than they used to be after a run or a game of tennis, a back or hip or knee that is a little troublesome, subtle changes in the way the stomach handles food or the colon handles elimination. Perhaps, we don't bounce out of bed quite as early, or we are a little more dependent on the pharmacy than we used to be. The journey is beginning and it involves a great deal of change. The good news is that if you don't resist, you can actually find a great deal of peace of mind and contentment in the present moment. And what can help you to focus your attention in present time and learn to catch and root out resistance is the skillful means you learn from the yoga methodology outlined in this book.

You may ask, "And just how is yoga going to help me get healthier and happier? How can I embrace change and be more comfortable with what is? How can I accept the course of my life and learn to be content and joyful in this moment — and just exactly how is this yoga business going to help me get *there*?" Turn the page.

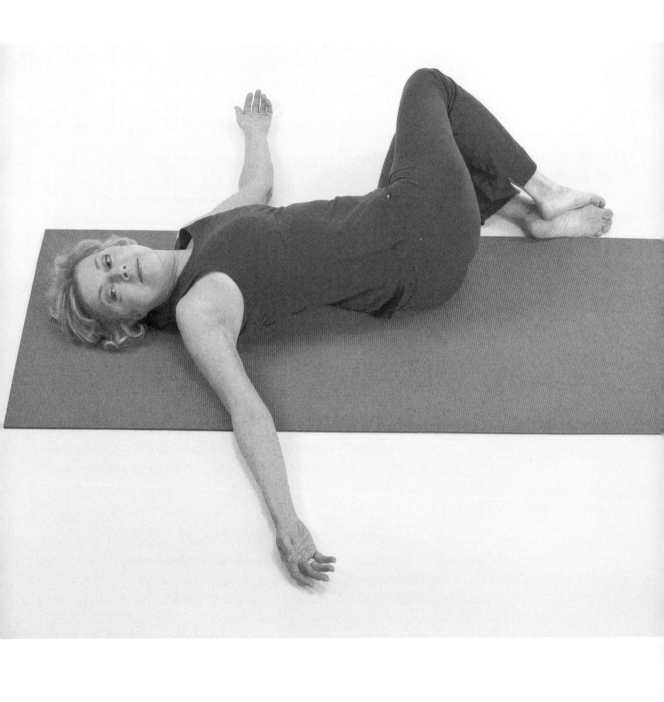

Chapter 2 **REST OR RUN?**

Every Moment Is a Choice

We are at a critical time in the evolution of the human species and I happen to think that is why yoga has appeared in the West as a method of personal growth, why more and more people are examining yoga, and probably why I'm writing this book on yoga now.

We are collectively looking for a map which will lead us out of the morass. The ancient methodology of classical yoga, which is the foundation for all the teachings in *Boomer Yoga*, is a trail map through the tangle. It was a practical guide for those seeking health and happiness two thousand years ago and, miraculously, it still is today. It shows us a way to live confidently and fearlessly in a world of constant change, to understand the ups and downs of life, and to maintain equipoise in the midst of the storms.

Yoga starts, for most of us, with what is called *asana* (pronounced "ah - sana"). Remember, the Sanskrit word *asana* refers to the practice of the yoga postures and at first glance it seems like just a little exercise. If we are tight, from life or a life of athletics, it might be a little difficult when we start out, but it feels good to stretch and sweat, so we persevere. If we continue to practice, the mental

training-tools that accompany this seemingly innocuous "exercise" teach us to focus and pay attention. However, unlike many other forms of exercise, this isn't a mindless activity. When we go to yoga class, our teachers tell us to listen to our breath, to hold a steady gaze, and to pay attention to our physical alignment, all of which sets us up to pay attention to the present moment. And this is the key, this is where the secret lies to the change that has just begun in our bodies and our minds.

What happens from this attentiveness training? It changes us — for the better. There is no other way to say it. The good news is that there is a way to have a nice little "yoga workout" as well as gain awareness, be happier, stay healthy longer, and take greater control over the course of your life and your health. How in the world does that happen?

The focus on mindfulness brings us into the only reality that there is, the NOW — and gets us out of our endless mental chatter and activity of plans, lists, and uncertainties about our escapades of yesterday and tomorrow. So what is so good about that? It feels good! For the hour that we have been in our yoga class, or practicing on our own at home with

THE YOGA CODE

In all the workshops I lead across the country, I ask the same question, "How many of you feel yoga has changed your life?" Everyone raises his or her hand. Yoga transforms us. How does it do that? Well, I like to say it's the *mystery of the methodology*. It's in the doing that the change happens. You can't explain it, you can't define it, you can only feel it — you become more aware, more conscious, and more compassionate. You start with *asana*, the practice of the yoga postures, and you learn at the most fundamental level to pay attention. That's the Yoga Code in a nutshell. Pay attention, make an effort to keep your mind steady, and watch what happens.

this book, we've been "here," and pretty much not worrying about our troubles, our finances, our regrets, our fears, our families, and so on. We've had a moment of peacefulness, of what we could call *aware presence*, or really being in touch with ourselves and the world around us. And after a few months of practicing we actually begin to notice the changes occurring, and we slowly start to realize that just by doing this yoga stuff we are moving towards a calmer, more centered, more content place in our lives. So does that make us passive? Less active? Less involved? Less passionate? Not at all. On the contrary, we are more present, more mindful, and more filled with wonder and appreciation for our life and our gifts. Really!

Classical yoga is a methodology that has re-surfaced and become popular at this time because, as I mentioned above, I believe it to be a roadmap out of the disarray and chaos we have created here on Earth. As I mentioned in chapter 1, this brilliant system, which we will explore in *Boomer Yoga*, is

from an ancient Sanskrit text that is over two thousand years old, entitled *The Yoga Sutra*, and was compiled by a sage and yogi named Patanjali. Around 2200 years ago, influenced by the prevalent teachings of Buddha, who had just left his lifetime on Earth a few hundred years earlier, Patanjali went around and collected all the lessons and principles of yoga, and put them into an incredibly logical, well-organized set of instructions for spiritual growth and personal health and evolution.

This collection became known as *The Yoga Sutra* and the system it describes is called classical or *raja* (royal) yoga, or *astanga* yoga. *Astanga* comes from the two words — *ashto*, or "eight," and *anga*, or "limb" — and the established reference to the word should not be confused with the currently popular and athletic form of yoga, also called *ashtanga*, that teaches a specific series of postures.

This classical system describes a path comprised of eight parts, or what yoga calls "limbs." These progress from basic fundamental and physical levels of training like the practice of *asana* (third limb), to increasingly subtle forms of training, like *pranayama* (fourth limb) and meditation (seventh limb). It is completely astonishing to me that this methodology is still so relevant now! But apparently, ever since Patanjali pulled it all together into a Yoga Code-type document, it has offered a way for people to be healthy and happy and get unstuck from the mud. If you come up with a way out of the mud, I don't think it matters so much whether it is now or two thousand years ago. If it works, let's keep it.

Reading *The Yoga Sutra* isn't like reading your average how-to book. It starts out giving the most esoteric aspect of the teaching first, but then goes on to give us a very practical method for really getting to know ourselves. The instructions, though, are buried in short, terse *sutras*, or aphorisms, which require translation and interpretation. There are dozens and dozens of translations available today, but they aren't easy to read. I've been studying *The Yoga Sutra* since the early '80s and only just now am I beginning to decipher some of the "heavier" messages! And I hope to pass these profound messages along to you in the ensuing chapters. But first, let's start with the basics.

We start with *asana*. The *asana* part of yoga practice is simply about developing good architecture — constructing a strong foundation, opening up tight spaces, awakening dead areas, restoring shut-down compartments

and blocked passageways in and out of the organs, and bringing in nutrition and healing energy via improved circulation of blood and intracellular fluid. *Asana* is practical — that's why it comes first in our training, even though it is not mentioned until Book 2 in the actual *Yoga Sutra*. However, it is traditional to begin the study of yoga with the practice of *asana*, as it is the portal into the more profound aspects of the yoga methodology.

We start with a very scientific system of engineering, constructing an architecturally sound foundation for our beautiful temple — which houses us — in which to carry on our activities. This requires a little work on our part: we need to pay attention to detail, we need to learn to focus, and to recognize where we need restoration and renovation. We need to build a clean and stable groundwork for the rest of our structure to stand and flourish. Once that is accomplished, we can move on, if we are interested, to the deeper, more spiritual, and mystical aspects of yoga.

Yes, this tangible set of instructions that begins with the practical teaching of *asana* will eventually lead you to the experience of yoga itself, which is a mystical experience, and cannot be described or explained. In order to experience yoga, you have to start doing yoga! Reading about yoga, wearing yoga clothes, hanging out with yogis, won't bring about much of anything. Sorry, nope, you gotta do it. And that begins with chapter 3 — the practice of *asana*.

And if you do it, the good news is that the rewards come fairly early — just in the "doing" of the practice, whether it is the practice of the postures or the practice of meditation, you will begin to notice change fairly quickly. I know this sounds a little corny, but how quickly depends on — you! Even *The Yoga Sutra* confirms (Book 1, Sutra 21) this by saying that to the keen and intent practitioner— the goal sits near by, waiting! You don't need to slog through eight to ten years of bending and binding and sitting and sweating before the change begins to occur! And you don't need to have a *pranayama* or meditation practice (chapters 7 and 8) to start being happier! You will see. The physical changes are apparent.

The mental and emotional changes are a little less obvious but evident nonetheless. Your desire to eat food that doesn't support your well-being, to chase unhealthy habits and practices, to be around negative people, just kind of slowly falls away. But all this good stuff depends on one thing — that you really do practice.

EVOLUTION OR EXTINCTION

If we could just step out of our existence, and look at ourselves — over the whole range of our evolution — as if we were looking at the history of another species and their environment, we would we horrified by the frightening picture we'd observe. With species extinction, global warming, out-of-control population growth, radical climate change, tribal warfare, the spread of poverty, massive deforestation, and desecration of the planet, the pressure on us as a species is phenomenal. You can feel it. And it's front-and-center news. We need help.

What happens when any species undergoes enormous environmental pressure? According to a number of scientists, including mathematical cosmologist and totally cool guy, Brian Swimme of the California Institute of Integral Studies, the major crisis we are facing is that we are smack in the middle of a mass extinction — the same as the one that happened sixty-five million years ago, when the dinosaurs got wiped off the Earth by a meteorite. Twenty-five thousand species are going extinct every year. He says, "We happen to be in that moment when the worst thing that's happened to the Earth in sixty-five million years is happening now. That's number one. Number two, we are causing it. Number three, we're not aware of it." Well, maybe we can't see it quite so clearly because we are smack in the middle of it — it's hard to get perspective.

Any one of these issues alone could precipitate a catastrophic change. And given that each of them feeds on and is fed by the others, how can we separate them? So overpopulation, climate change, non-sustainability, water quality, pollution, etc., combine to become this huge burgeoning encumbrance that turns back into itself and amplifies itself like a billowing tornado. Any species undergoing this type of environmental pressure has only a few choices — two to be precise — evolution or extinction. A species must mutate and/or transform itself to adapt to the changing environment or it will die off.

THE BIG WAKE-UP CALL

So, will we survive or will we die off? What will happen? Funny thing, the planet might possibly be fine, no matter what we do. Supposedly, we're due for another Ice Age, global warming or no global warming, in about thirty to fifty thousand years. But based on the way things are going, we can't really predict that with any certainty. Climate change is a normal, natural thing. And there are instances when it can be very welcome — like ten thousand years ago, when the last Ice Age ended and we transitioned to the current, more hospitable (to us anyway) climate. But we have accelerated the pace of natural climate change so our planet is in peril and we, and the rest of the Earth's inhabitants, are the ones who are vulnerable.

Why is that? Well, for many of us, things seem to be changing rapidly "out there." But in our small, fragmented corner of the world that we have carved for ourselves, once we get comfortable we work so hard to keep the illusion of status quo that nothing appears to change. We work hard to keep our immediate environment the same. We form our self-identities by the things and thoughts and world views we accumulate. Species disappearing? Why, whatever does that mean? Some frog in the rainforest is no more? Some bug in the Everglades has disappeared? It seems distant, not especially relevant to us. Well, those days are over. What in the world makes us think that if so many species are dying off, that we are somehow impervious to this extinction? Our health as a species depends on biodiversity.

As recently as early 2008, the seriousness of the environmental situation had not really hit Main Street. Many of us were still thinking, "What's the problem? I'm not feeling the effects. I still have my kids, my back yard, my bank account, my car, my bottled water from Fiji and my bananas in winter, my vacation, and my gas barbeque. Wal-Mart and Target and Best Buy have more offerings of 'stuff' every year, not less. What could possibly be missing? A few species? What's the big deal?"

But by the summer of 2008 the entire species of the planet began to receive a huge wake-up call and it wasn't until the catastrophic economic failure hit us with both barrels in the fall of that year that we began, as a tribe, to pay attention. Our backyards were in turmoil. Many of us lost our backyards altogether. Our cars cost a fortune to put on the road. Our retirement was up in smoke. Now it was not just the environment, but our global economic structure that was collapsing. All those things we counted on not to change — our bank account, our retirement, our investments, our pension, even our job — were proving to be not all that secure. From Middle America to the Coasts and back, people were reeling with the speed of change and the fears that accompanied it. We used to think that if we worked for Bell Telephone or Exxon or General Motors or General Electric or whomever, that they would take care of us forever. We'd have a pension, a plan for leaving our profession, and a happy home in the lush green acres of retirement. But where are those assurances now?

We are seeing that not only can our employers not guarantee us safety and security, but neither can our government leaders nor our religious leaders. Even our families can't promise to provide for us in our later years, as we see more of the elderly being placed in nursing homes and home-care "facilities." rather than living with their adult children. We are discovering that things we thought were permanent, are not — and never were.

Even our wilderness, our supply of renewable energy, and our prosperity as a nation cannot provide the permanent security we thought they might. As long as we try and work out our internal security, and ultimately, our happiness, through someone or something that is external to ourselves — our spouse or partner, our kids, our profession, our acquisitions — we will be disappointed over and over again. Why? Because we are looking for security — which we often equate with a state of changelessness — and all the things we are looking to provide that security are part of the world of form (the material world), or what in Sanskrit is called *prakriti*. But the very nature of the world of form is to change constantly, and therefore cannot guarantee any type of security.

And when things change, we become uncomfortable. Actually it's not too bad if things change for the "better," although that is stressful too. But if the change appears to bring uncertainty or loss or pain, whooee, well then, we surely don't want that. What we want is a lifetime guarantee of eternal bliss. But we are bound to be disappointed because that isn't the nature of the world of form! The world is actually half heaven and half hell, half pleasure and half pain, half gain and half loss. We may only want to hang out with what we perceive to be the "good" half, but like it or not, we get the whole shebang.

Our dependency on the outside world to be stable, unchanging, and comfortable will lead us to disillusionment and much suffering, as sooner or later, we are all forced to learn. If we don't learn it easily with a few nudges the first couple times around, then life gives us a big shove and the lessons become more intense until we finally do learn it. This seems to be what's going on for us as a species right now. Wham! says the Universe. Take that. People don't think conditions are serious? Okay, let's give them a little lesson in the eventual results of unmitigated greed and show how, by pulling the bottom out of economic stability, we can slow the negative effects on the environment. People will spend less, consume less, recycle more, and downsize in general.

I happen to think that this recent economic calamity — as well as all the storms, from meteorological to cultural — is a karmic reaction to our overall disregard for one another and our planet. It is caused by what in yoga is called *parigraha*, or acquisitiveness, greediness. Our collective greed has nearly taken us over as a species — and now we've received a global wake-up call. Rise and shine.

CHANGE IS INEVITABLE

Many of us were shocked into wakefulness on the state of our environment by Al Gore's documentary film, *An Inconvenient Truth*, which I saw in 2006. This Academy Award-winning documentary graphically brought home for many people the urgency of the global warming crisis. The reality of climate change and its impact on life on this planet hit me when I was in Alaska teaching yoga in the summer of 2007. I spent one cold rainy day heading up 20 Mile Glacier River in Chugach National Park. Not many people navigate this river by boat in the best of weather, and on this day, it was pretty miserable, so there were only a few other boats on the water and they were all relatively far downstream from the source of the river — the glacier — puttering around and trying to look like they were actually doing something.

Of the few tourists that make it all the way upriver to 20 Mile River Lake, most go by plane, as not many boats are equipped and not many drivers experienced enough to navigate the fast-running, shallow waters. The only type of boat that can make it upriver is a jet boat, which draws only about three to four inches of water when it's under power, and in order to stay that high the boat has to go at top speed, dodging the logs and trees and

rocks sticking out everywhere.

So imagine: a swift, shallow, boulder-strewn, obstacle course of a river, and a boat that has to go like hell in order to navigate it. Our driver, Andy Morrison of Alaska Backcountry Access was a very calm, cool, and collected fellow and the epitome of confidence. It's a good thing. Because everyone else I'd talked to prior to the trip had me convinced that if I made it through this journey without being jettisoned out of the boat, impaled on a tree trunk, or chased back to Anchorage by a grizzly, I'd be among a very select group of travelers who had made it to the 20 Mile Glacier and lived to write about it. Andy had pioneered guiding tours up this river for ten years and was an awesome driver. The ride itself was a white-knuckle experience, but not nearly as terrifying or death-defying as I'd been led to believe. It was, in fact, exhilarating, kind of like Category 5 whitewater kayaking, except in a boat. We stopped a few times and floated to watch bald eagles fish, and to watch them watch us, then hit the ground, errr, I mean the water, running again. When we entered the lake, I was totally unprepared for what I saw before me.

It was cold, maybe thirty-five degrees and raining. The lake was totally socked in with icy vapor. The frosty mist was slowly expanding up and out, covering the water like a ghostly apparition. We cut the engine and just floated. Appearing out of the vapor, like phantom spirits, enormous chunks of ancient frozen water materialized right before my eyes. They were an incredible blue, as unspeakable as the deepest reaches of space — a blue like nothing I had ever seen. It was deadly silent, except for one sound, the sound of dripping. We floated beyond time and space. No one said a word. The power of the silence just overwhelmed all six or seven of us in the boat.

Then, as we floated closer to the middle of the lake, there came forth from the womb of the Earth the most enormous apparition — rising up out of the water — blue into the depths of the soul, the mother of our journey, the mother of everyone's journey, the original Goddess, beckoning to me, smiling, saying, Yes, we are here. This massive chunk of ice had broken free from the glacier and was floating, an iceberg in the lake. I began to cry. She cried. We cried together. We went closer and I touched her. I knew her from thousands of lifetimes ago. We both knew in that moment — nothing in the world of form is permanent.

Eventually we powered up the boat and slowly made our way up to the edge of the glacier, at a place where it flattened out into the water. I just knew I had to hold this ancient being in my arms. I climbed out, picking my way across ice and exposed bits of rock and sediment. I stood on the glacier and listened to it melt. Drip, drip, drip. The glacier spoke to me. And I don't mean that figuratively. The glaciers are alive. The water dripping into my hands, as I gently cupped them under a glacial overhang, was alive — returning to its form as water for the very first time in ten thousand years. Hydrogen atoms — billions of years old — were humming with the primordial sound of Om. The immensity of what I was witnessing, of what I was holding in my hands, was overpowering. I sat on the glacier and cried again. I cried for myself, my own mortality (the Great Illusion), for the illusion of permanence in form, for all of time, for all of life, for all of us. It was as if the face of God melted into my hands and spoke to me. Another moment of boundlessness. I was the water, the glacier, the eternal movement of the Universe from particle into wave, wave into particle. Form becoming emptiness, emptiness becoming form.

It was an extraordinary moment that helped me to really understand the meaning of impermanence. Nothing is still. Every single atom in this spacious, far-reaching universe of ours is moving, shifting, realigning its place in the cosmos — coming and going, becoming manifest, then unmanifest, then manifest again. Change is inevitable. It happens no matter what we do. Some change we can control, some not. We can mold, direct, and influence the direction of our lives. But we cannot hold back change. Are the glaciers melting simply because it is their time to melt? Are we accelerating the process as a species through our lifestyle? Can we influence the rate of change? And then I got back into the jetboat and headed back down the river with everyone else, snapping pictures and looking forward to dinner at a nice restaurant in Anchorage.

HOW CAN YOGA HELP ME?

Global warming (or overpopulation, or species extinction, or pollution) has a lot more to do with our desire as a species not to own up to our greediness, our "species-ism," our predatory way of wiping out other species, our arrogance about our position on the food chain, our cultural Western obsession with stuff and accumulating wealth, than it does with any "natural" cycle. We are nudging the thermostat and there will be repercussions.

So, how can we look at what is going on and keep on doing what we are doing? Well, either we aren't seeing or we are seeing but just ignoring. Isn't that completely crazy? Well, over the past few years, it seems that more and more of us are not willing to keep on doing what we've been doing. We are looking for transformation, whether we totally know it or not. We are ready to change. We are being forced to change. And I think that is why so many of us are turning to yoga and possibly even why you bought this book. Think about it. Are you just looking for a workout? Or are you looking for something a little deeper, a little more profound? Yoga is one path that's available today to people of all ages, religions, and cultures, that can lead to an essential sense of total well-being. It's a powerful tool for transformation. Just follow the instructions and practice in this book.

You may be completely new to yoga, but if you commit to the work, which begins with *asana*, an easy forty minutes a day, three or four days a week, you will move toward happiness and contentment. And even if you have done yoga, or have been doing it for years, unless you are a student of mine you haven't done it in this way. But no matter what yoga you do, if it is authentic practice, the change comes. Ask anyone you know who has been doing yoga for some time. Their yoga practice has helped them to be stronger, to see more clearly, to be more community-minded, to be happier and more centered no matter what is happening on Wall Street, and to gain greater awareness of the connectedness of all beings and to see that we are all in this together!

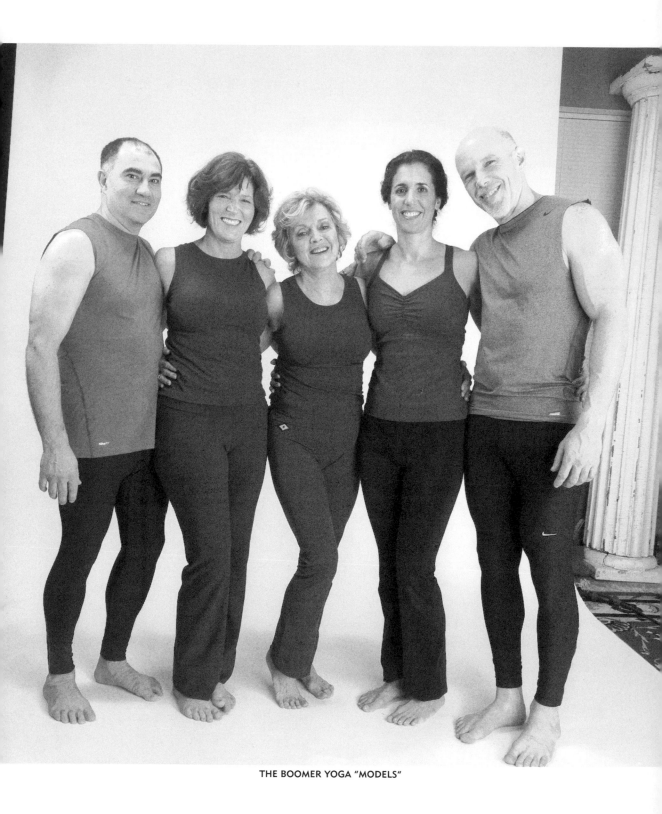

THE BOOMER YOGA "MODELS"

Chapter 3 BUILDING THE FIRE

Turning Up the Heat

As I look back over the years at the many times I have softened, toughened, changed, modified, adjusted, and reworked my practices to accommodate the ever-changing world of *prakriti* (form), I realize how much that whole process has taught me about "impermanence." In the cases when I was resistant to the change, which generally went hand in hand with not fully paying attention and not seeing the necessity to "adjust" voluntarily, the Universe generally reached out and helped me to "see" the need to make a small modification!

All those many experiences and "lifetimes" have really helped me to see what a shifting, malleable thing this life is, and that just when we think we are all set for clear sailing, boom, a storm appears out of nowhere. We really do have to be able to reset our course at a moment's notice. One way or another we learn through childhood how to navigate the rough waters, with teachers, mentors, and role models to help us set our path. In the end we realize that our journey is our own — based on our unique *karma*, experiences, *samskara* (energetic impressions), preferences, and previous lifetimes. Our passage is unlike any other and we can only depend on our

teachers and mentors to offer guidance, but not to take the journey for us. The actual moving forward has to come from within.

What connects us all is the desire to evolve, to go deeper, and to know who we truly are — beyond conditioned thought, beyond social conditioning, beyond our world views. But what eventually takes us to this realization is an experience that is matchless. We are connected by a universal desire to evolve, but each of us must find our own distinctive path. So it follows that each of our yoga paths will be distinctive as well. Because I have been practicing for so long and teaching for so many years, I've had the opportunity to build *asana* practices, the place most people start their practice of yoga, for literally tens of thousands of people. Every single practice has been slightly different just based on the fact that every single individual is different.

I will give a number of options throughout the book as to what you can do to modify your *asana* routine. If, like me, you have had injuries or if you have medical conditions that limit your abilities, you will still be able to do these postures one way or another. But it will require a bit of experimentation on your part. Perhaps you have high blood pressure, or high cholesterol, or osteoarthritis, or you may have had knee or shoulder surgery, or are going through menopause. Or maybe you have prostate issues, or irritable bowel syndrome, or are recovering from cancer. Lord, there are nearly an infinite number of challenges that crop up as we get older, and many ways in which we fall out of wellness, but each condition manifests differently in every individual. So although we will work through a basic routine in this book, there will be choices and options, not only for the practice of *asana* in chapters 3–6, but for the practice of breath work and meditation in the chapters that follow.

But one thing is important for all of us to know despite our differences in age, health, and well-being: Yoga is supposed to help. It is, in all its forms, a therapeutic system, and can be healing and helpful for all of the conditions mentioned above, as well as many others. Today there is greater cooperation between the traditional, medical field and the alternative systems of healing from around the world. The combined knowledge of the best of the Western and Eastern traditions has come to be known as "integrative medicine." More and more, I find in my travels, people telling me about how their physicians have recommended they start yoga. It is encouraging to see, for those of us who have been practicing and studying yoga for decades, that it has begun to be accepted by the medical world as a legitimate aid to stress reduction, wellness, and healing.

But this is not only a book about how yoga can help people suffering specifically from say, fibromyalgia or rheumatoid arthritis. There are many different yoga *asana* styles out there that can be helpful for a variety of illnesses and injuries. Some methods are strong, some are softer, some are more active, some are more restorative, some are more difficult, some are easier. Since each individual and yoga style is different, the degree of beneficial effects will vary. *Boomer Yoga* presents a "middle path" and a "way in" to the world of yoga. It is both steady and comfortable, active and restorative, and yes, at times, it will be difficult — but it will also become easier. This is a doable system that most folks can try and can understand. Once we are in, and actually "practicing," we can begin to make choices for ourselves and to understand the kind of work we need to do to either get well or stay well.

WHAT TO EXPECT

If I were just starting out in yoga now, or looking to deepen an existing interest that consists of, say attending a class or two a week, I would first want to develop an *asana* practice that is malleable enough to change and mature with my interests and abilities. I would want something *soft* enough to be able to actually *do* but *hard* enough to challenge and strengthen my body and mind, and *disciplined* enough to guide me toward concentration and meditation.

All yoga, in its many layers, is yoga therapy, or should be. Yoga therapy isn't just something

HEATIN' UP OR CHILLIN' OUT

Whether you are just starting out with yoga, stepping up to a stronger practice, stepping down to a more structured, less frenetic system of exercise, or simply in need of some yoga therapy, this "boomer yoga" routine is ordered enough to provide structure, yet flexible enough to provide exactly what your mind and body need. As I mentioned above, I'll give a variety of choices for most of the postures in the successive chapters. As you get the hang of it, you'll find that you are making modifications for yourself and developing your own personal practice based on preference and aptitude. I've found over the years that this practice is what I call *adaptogenic*; that is, if I'm too cool or lethargic and metabolically challenged, it revs up the engines and heats me up. Conversely, if I'm too amped up or stressed out, it calms me down and chills me out.

you seek out if you are ill or injured. The therapeutic element should be integral to your practice. Your practice should help to keep your back from hurting and your body flexible, to help you to avoid unnecessary surgery. For example, as we age, our joints, organs, muscles, and bones all become subject to a variety of degenerative influences. So our practice needs to work as a system of detoxification, a way to flush toxins and keep the immune system strong and fully engaged, and the joints supple and lubricated. The more *rajasic* (active) of the *asana* systems are specifically designed to do this through sweating and squeezing out pollutants, and God knows we've got plenty of them in our environment in today's world.

I remember when I first started teaching my power yoga method in 1980 in New York City people who came were amazed after class that you can sweat while you are doing yoga. Big tough football players and weight lifters would often exclaim after class, "Oh my God, that's the hardest thing I've ever done." Well it was *hard* for them because they were tight — so they struggled and grunted and, naturally, sweat a lot. Generally we associate sweating with huffing and puffing and working hard. Eventually though, in yoga we learn to work hard, but also to work smart. The breath is even, powerful, and controlled, not panting. The heart rate is even and steady, not pounding. We are statically contracting muscles, and focusing on those contractions — it isn't a stretch class. Those strong, conscious contractions are different from the dynamic contractions of running or biking that build lactic acid (*asana* practice does not). The contractions, along with two other yoga techniques — one, a special breathing method and the other, internal muscular contractions to move energy and create heat — help to keep the sweating mechanism turned on, and wring the toxins out of the muscles, ligaments, and tendons.

We begin with training the body and end, if

there is such a thing, with the realization that all along we have been training the mind as well. The practice we are going to build here is based on a methodology, an ancient set of instructions that will take us from gross levels of awareness to levels subtle beyond gossamer. Because we have been learning to pay attention with ever-increasing vigilance, our awareness deepens and our focus shifts from simply seeing what is right under our nose to seeing with greater vision and sensitivity.

So let's begin and look at how we can layout an *asana* practice for ourselves that is both hard and soft: hard enough to push the envelope a bit and soft enough to actually do and enjoy! The practice has lots of malleability in it. You will make choices — intelligent ones, I know — about which path is best for you. Saddle up, here we go!

TRIBUTE TO THE SUN

The sun held a central place in the life and thought of ancient India, as in most ancient and indigenous cultures. Going back thousands of years, the day almost always began — all over the planet — with the worship of the sun. I am certainly not an expert on the following cultures, but it seems to me that the Mayans, the Incas, the Aztecs, the Native Americans, the Eskimos, the Druids, the Romans, the Greeks, and I'm sure dozens of others, all had sun temples and sun deities. The sun was the symbol of the great light that the human soul longed to find — whether consciously or not — within. Just think about the importance of the sun in our own culture. Well, for starters, without it we wouldn't be here.

So it is no surprise that a short sequence of movements called the Sun Salutation (from the Sanskrit *Surya Namaskar*, or literally "obeisance to the sun") is the way most yoga *asana* methods begin their practice. In my opinion, there really isn't a better way to start. I feel that nothing else does quite as good a job of warming up the body for a strong *asana* practice. The Sun Salutation serves as a foundation for the subsequent postures and is just about a complete workout in itself as it loosens and heats up every joint and corner of the body.

Many yoga schools and traditions use one or another adaptation of the Sun Salutation as the basic warm-up for their classes and practices. I've been doing Sun Salutations — in slightly different variations — as part of every *asana* practice I've ever done. I did them in the '70s, the '80s, the '90s, and am still doing them today. Over the years, I've modified them for my own practice to accommodate a broken leg, carpal tunnel syndrome, a torn rotator cuff muscle, osteoarthritis in a hip, and a variety of shoulder injuries, sprained ankles, and lower back strain. I've taught them to people of all ages, to all types of athletes, to people with all kinds of limitations and restrictions and illness, to paraplegics, quadriplegics, blind persons, and people in wheelchairs. I just speak with them and tune into what they can do, and then I create a modified program that will work for them. The great thing is that everyone can do the breathing — Up Dog, Down Dog, extend, flex, breathe — yes!

DETOXING

The particular system of *asana* practice described in this book is what in yoga is called a form of *tapas*, or *detoxification*. The word tapas literally means "to burn." The idea is that you use the work to start an internal fire, which then in turn burns impurities and clears toxins from the body, through squeezing, sweating, and breathing.

The Sun Salutation we are going to work with here is a sequence of nine positions and each position or movement flows from one to the next. It is performed, once learned, as a fluid sort of dance with one breath accompanying each move, and is generally repeated several times. The idea is to use this work to warm up for the rest of your practice. Hopefully, by the time you finish doing the repetitions you will have broken into a sweat. That's the idea.

A FEW THINGS TO KNOW

First of all, if you can, it's best to do your *asana* practice in the morning because it really sets you up for the day. According to my personal yoga polls, people report it gets them grounded, centered, loosened up, and just makes the rest of the day go easier. But lots of people can't do that — you've got kids to get to school, or you have to get yourself to work, or you have a run to get in, or a family to tend to — it can be tough. My husband Thom and I spent twenty-two years in New York City teaching classes through the New York Road Runners Club on Monday and Wednesday nights to over 100,000 folks who couldn't do their yoga in the morning. So do the best you can — and get this in whenever you can. But keep in mind, you

can't do this on a full stomach or after a beer and pizza. I mean you *can*, of course, but use your head. It's best on an empty stomach, or with just a banana or a piece of fruit or toast, or a cup of coffee or tea. A full stomach can cause nausea, sleepiness, or mindlessness. You don't want to be absent mentally when you're practicing or learning yoga — you want complete attention. So, bottom line, do it in the morning if you can, or if not, before lunch (while you're in your office — get out your mat — you only need eighteen square feet) or after work before dinner.

Personally, I'm too exhausted at night to do *asana* or much of anything after about 6:00 p.m., except read and eat dinner. I go to bed by 9:00 or 9:30 p.m. and get up at 5:30 a.m. I'm a full-on morning person and go roaring through a walk or yoga *asana* or breathing exercises or a bike ride early in the day. But that's me. You could be a night owl — in which case you'll be perfectly happy doing yoga at 7:00 p.m. and eating your dinner at 9:00 p.m.

Next, you've got to be hydrated. That means you need to drink water — plenty of it — before you practice. Especially if you have high blood pressure or high cholesterol, you need to be well hydrated. In fact, you need to drink a boat load of water as a matter of course, even if you're in the best of health. Oh yes, I know there is all this hoopla and recent research about drinking too much water and blah blah, and I'm sure it can happen that people drink too much and develop some horrid condition, but personally I haven't ever seen this happen. Drink between 32 and 64 ounces a day — depending on what you are doing and how much you are sweating. My grandma always said eight glasses a day — sounds good to me. I am sure we have all heard some health-care professional tell us that we need to drink sufficient amounts of water. This practice is designed to make you sweat, unless you unwisely decide to practice in an air conditioned house or gym. So drink plenty of water before you practice so that you derive the benefit of the practice as *tapas*.

Try to keep distractions to a dull roar. The other morning I went to teach a private yoga class to a client in an enormous house here in East Hampton. There were quite a few house guests out for the weekend and they were spread out all over the place. A number of people wanted to take the class, and they all wanted to practice out on the lawn. An entire landscaping crew was in attendance as well — mowing, raking, blowing, and weed whacking. There were about seven young teenage girls leaping in and out of the pool with gay abandon, and the neighbors were preparing for a party later that night, and their band for the evening was warming up. People were wandering in and out of the house, chewing on bacon and lugging bagels laden with cream cheese, looking for mats and wanting to join in. As I

struggled to find some order and began to call out the cadence for the Sun Salutations, I just broke up laughing. It was crazy!

We all have to deal with distractions — they are part of life. Whether they are internal (such as the constant stream of conditioned thought produced by our minds), or external (something we see or hear that captures our attention), as we learn to focus and direct our attention, the distractions become less attractive. We're able to let the interfering thought pass; we're not drawn in by the external sight or sound. But sometimes a distraction is just too big to ignore. I joke around with my students and say, "Look, if a whole herd of elephants run through here, I don't want to see anyone blink."

Just a few mornings ago, I was working with another yoga client here in town. He is a super-bright, high-powered, Type A personality with high blood pressure who wants to get the practice *right* immediately. In the beginning, he was constantly distracted by his own mind. But I'd been teaching this fellow for several weeks and he was really beginning to settle down, get better with his concentration, and go for longer periods of time without opening his mouth to ask a question. But the other morning, just as he was all warmed up, sweating, breathing, and preparing to "bind" in a posture (which basically means wrapping oneself up in a posture, but in a good way — not necessarily pretzel-like) he took a call from his mother. Uh, it didn't go well after that. So, when you're planning to practice, see if you can pick a time when anticipated disturbances can be kept to a minimum.

VICTORY BREATH:
Learning *Ujjayi* Breathing

There is a unique form of breathing that accompanies this yoga practice, which some of you may already be familiar with, called *ujjayi* (pronounced "u'jai'yee") breathing. The Sanskrit word *ujjayi* means "expand into victory" so *ujjayi* is often called "victory breath." This is hands-down an incredible and powerfully therapeutic technique that everyone in the world should learn — whether or not they ever do *asana*. It can be used in all conditions to create heat, relax, get present, chill out, train the mind in concentration, and develop control of the breath.

Ujjayi breath is done with the mouth closed — both on the inhale and the exhale. The idea is to keep your mouth shut for the entire duration of your practice, the premise being that every time you open your mouth, you lose *prana* or energy. The breathing technique itself, when done correctly, creates a sound — which happens as a result of a conscious, but very slight, constriction of the muscles in the throat — just above the vocal cords. You are actually already familiar with how to do this as it happens automatically every time you whisper. As you talk, that sort of raspy sound is made as air flows across the vocal cords. This happens as a result of a narrowing of the passageway of the throat. Volume decreases, velocity increases (remember high school physics?).

To learn to do *ujjayi* breathing, whisper an "ahhhh" sound out loud with your mouth open. Or else imagine that you are using your breath to fog your glasses for cleaning — same idea. Both of these things require that you constrict your throat slightly. *Ujjayi* breathing requires exactly the same tightening, only it's done with the mouth closed. To get the hang of it, whisper "ahhhh" out loud again, then do the same thing with your mouth closed, both on the inhale and the exhale. The exhale will be easier at first. If you feel like you are gagging, or clearing your throat, you are working a little too hard. If there is no sound, as there is when you whisper "ahhhh" with your mouth open, you don't have it yet.

You've got to get this breathing technique before you start in order for your practice to be *yoga*. Practice this — you'll get it.

BE CLEAN, GET A MAT, AND BREATHE

Be clean and orderly. Krishnamurti, one of the greatest philosophers and best-known spiritual teachers of the twentieth century, always used to say that you can't have an orderly mind in a disorderly environment. He wasn't referring to saints or great spiritual masters who could go out into the world's madness and maintain their equipoise. He was talking about the rest of us who need all the help we can get in developing a quiet mind and aware presence. That means an orderly physical environment, like clean clothes and clean body, simple nourishment, and an organized environment — plus an orderly state of mind. In yoga, this principle is called *saucha* and means purity; I'll talk more about it in chapter 7.

One more thing: you need a yoga mat — a good, non-slip mat that's not too thick. Not those old, overstuffed, slidey plastic things from the '70s. And don't rent a mat at the local yoga studio — unless you can take it home and wash it in your washing machine before and after you use it. That's like borrowing someone else's tennis shoes to play tennis. It's gross. Get your own. Yoga mats are ubiquitous. You can order them online from about a kabillion sources. There are lots that are green and bio-degradable, made from cotton and/or rubber. Don't buy one that is made from PVC (poly-vinyl chloride). They take 13,000 billion years to break down. Practice on a wood, tile, granite, marble, cement, or bamboo floor. That's the first choice. Carpet is okay but not preferable — it's too mushy and not great for your wrists or your balance. And *no air conditioning* — cold air defeats the whole purpose of the practice. If you don't like sweating, find something else to do with yourself.

You will need to master the technique of *ujjayi* breathing described in the sidebar on page 33. Practice it while showering, driving to work, riding on the subway, chopping carrots, playing with your kids, any time you think of it. The breath must be correct — mouth closed, with sound, in control. Without it, you're just doing exercise. This is not just regular breathing; this is a conscious breathing technique that you need to pay attention to in order to do. It trains you to focus your mind. Once you have learned the *ujjayi* technique, the next step will be to link this conscious breath to a movement in the *asana* practice. Every movement in the *asana* practice is linked to the *ujjayi* breath and accompanied by either an inhalation or an exhalation.

PREPARING FOR THE SUN SALUTATION

Stand at the end of your yoga mat. Bring your feet together, big toes touching. If balance is an issue for you, you can separate your heels a bit, or even move your feet apart slightly if you feel unsteady with them touching. But, if so, make sure they are perfectly parallel! Level the pelvis, by tucking the tailbone. Often, if we have a bit of a belly, our pelvis tips forward, the butt sticks out, and there is excess compression in the lower back. Really be mindful to drop the tailbone and balance the pelvic "bowl."

Lift the thighs, and lift the chest bone (the sternum), and pull the belly in. This starting posture is called Mountain Posture, or sometimes in class I refer to it as Attention Position. You will begin and end your practice in this position, and frequently return to it between most of the Standing Postures for the entire Standing sequence.

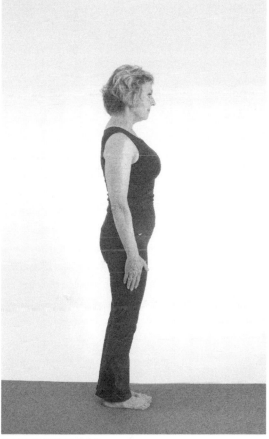

MOUNTAIN POSTURE

While in Mountain Posture, and before you dive into the Sun Salutation, take a moment to focus your eyes on a point in front of you. That means pick some little spot and look at it. Don't move your eyes, don't fidget. This "gaz-ing point" is called a *drishti* in yoga, and every posture has one. As you will see in the coming chapters, this point of focus for the eyes will change from posture to posture. What could you imagine the point of that might be? "Well, it keeps us from getting distracted and looking around," you might say. Yes! Good! That is correct. This is a bear of a discipline. It takes some people years and years to master it. They just can't resist looking around at whatever anyone else is doing (if they are in class) or noticing that there are dust particles under the couch or dog hairs on the floor (if they are at home). You'll need to stay focused, despite the distractions (and trust me, even if your kid or spouse or partner or dog or cat or neighbor doesn't interrupt, something or someone will!)

Before you dive in, take a moment to settle in and actually be there. Start your *ujjayi* breathing.

SUN SALUTATION — SURYA NAMASKARA (POSITIONS 1-9)

Each of the following nine positions will be completed on one inhalation or one exhalation. In other words, the breath should begin as you start each movement and end as you complete that movement.

NOTE: If this is difficult at first, put in an extra breath wherever necessary until you are able to move through the entire sequence controlling your breath as directed.

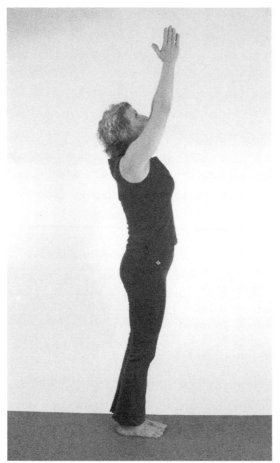

SUN SALUTATION POSITION 1

POSITION 1

Inhale as you bring your arms up over your head, with arms parallel or palms touching. It's okay if your arms are slightly off vertical.

Look up at your thumbs. This is your *drishti* or gazing point for this posture (photo above). If you have neck issues or it feels painful to look up, don't. In that case, look straight ahead. Stand straight up and down, don't lean back. If you have tight shoulders, you are going to want to lean back to get your arms

straight up. Don't lean back (especially if you have chronic lower back pain), as it tends to compress the lumbar spine (photo below). Instead, level your pelvis, drop your tailbone and pull your belly in. You want your ears, shoulders, hips, knees, and ankles all in one straight line. No curves backwards.

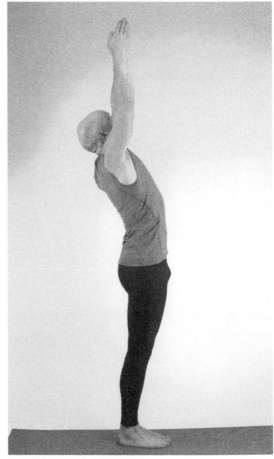

**SUN SALUTATION POSITION 1,
INCORRECT FORM**

If you're just starting out with your yoga practice and you're tight in the hamstrings or the hips, you should always bend your knees when you're bending over. This helps prevent back injury or strain. It's not wise or good for you to bend the back with straight legs unless your tailbone is the highest point of your back when you're bending over (photo below, right). This can be a little tricky to do. So get some help from someone in the house or ask a friend to stand next to you on the side. Bend over as far as you can with straight legs; then, as you are bending over, get them to put their hand on the highest point of your back. If it isn't the tailbone, then don't bend forward without bending your knees.

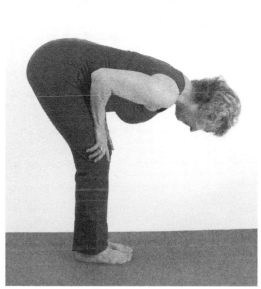

SUN SALUTATION POSITION 2

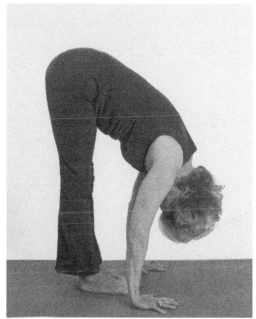

SUN SALUTATION POSITION 2, ADVANCED POSTURE

POSITION 2

Exhale as you bend forward and put your hands on your knees. Round the back gently and look down, so the *drishti* is down and back toward your navel (photo above, left). You will probably be tempted at some point to try and take your hands all the way to the floor, as I am doing in photo above, right. You can only do this safely if you have pretty flexible hamstrings and, if when you can bend over with straight legs, the highest point on your back is your tailbone at the base of your spine.

NOTE: Standing forward bending is contraindicated for persons with tight hamstrings or lower back pain or any kind of low back injury. The photo at right illustrates exactly what you don't want to do. You can see by looking at this photo, showing incorrect form, that if the backs of your legs are tight, it prevents you from bending all the way over. You can easily see why this isn't great for your back — gravity creates compression in the anterior (or front) portion of the spine, especially at the middle and lower back, as the back rounds forward.

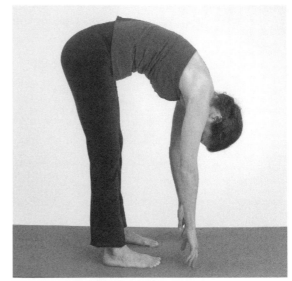

SUN SALUTATION POSITION 2, INCORRECT FORM

POSITION 3

Inhale as you arch your back and look up, keeping your hands on your bent knees. *Drishti* is up, so look up. If you are flexible enough to be working with your hands on the floor, the instructions are the same; lift your chest, look up.

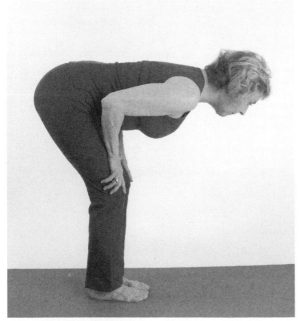

SUN SALUTATION POSITION 3

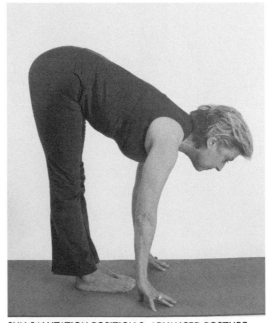

SUN SALUTATION POSITION 3, ADVANCED POSTURE

POSITION 4

Exhale as you drop down, take your hands to the floor, placing them directly under your shoulders and on either side of your feet while stepping all the way back to come into a straight or plank posture (below, top photo). Separate your feet hip-width apart.

Lower your knees to the floor, then lower your torso down into a push up position, keeping your torso — from the knees up — steel-straight and off the floor if you can.

Hold your elbows tucked in at your sides and upper arms parallel to the floor.

Keep your head in line with your spine. The *drishti* is out past the end of your nose (bottom photo).

Eventually this all happens on one exhalation: hands to floor, legs back, plank pose, knees down, and lower down into push up.

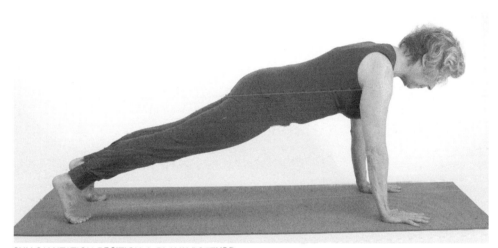

SUN SALUTATION POSITION 4, PLANK POSTURE

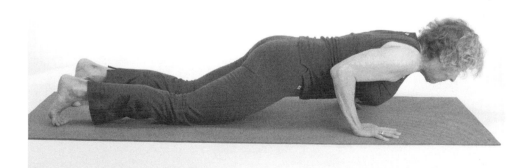

SUN SALUTATION POSITION 4

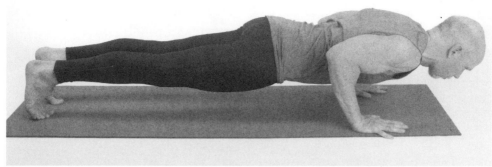

SUN SALUTATION POSITION 4, ADVANCED POSTURE

If you are strong enough to hold a push-up without sagging, then you can do the more advanced version where you don't need to put your knees down. Even if you are using your knees, eventually you will build up enough strength in the triceps so you won't need to put your knees down.

Shoulder injuries? You'll have to just work easy and see how it goes. Keep backing off until you can do the movement without stress or pain. Don't sag into your lower back, struggling to hold a push up — it stresses your lumbar spine and shoulders, plus it looks stupid and sloppy.

If you have limited plantar flexion (the ability to point your toes), both versions of Position 5 might be a little uncomfortable (arghhh!), so continue with the knees-down posture, until the tops of your feet stretch out a little. If you have lower back pain or injury, it is best to use the knees-down modification or skip the posture altogether.

The next two postures (Face Up Dog Posture and Face Down Dog Posture) are great if you have osteoporosis (or osteopenia) and the condition is manifesting in the upper thoracic spine (the portion of your spine roughly between your shoulders and the bottom of your rib cage) through excessive curvature. These postures, as well as all the Standing Postures, will help to reverse the degenerative tendency of this curve to increase as we get older, especially if our bones are weak. You might want to work to actually hold each position for 5 breaths.

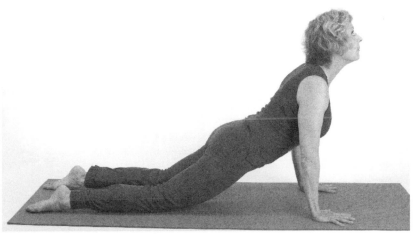

SUN SALUTATION POSITION 5, FACE UP DOG POSTURE

POSITION 5

Inhale as you change the position of your feet, so that your toes are pointed and the tops of your feet are flat on the floor. Keep your knees on the floor and your hands directly under your shoulders.

Press into your arms, and lift all the way up, straightening your arms, rolling the shoulders back, and arching slightly. Don't hang into your shoulders. Lift up! *Drishti* is straight out or slightly up (photo above). This posture is commonly called Face Up Dog Posture

If you would like to do a more challenging version of Position 5, push down into the tops of your feet and lift your knees off the floor. Keep the entire torso lifted off the floor. Look up. Don't sag into your lower back or shoulders. Use the shoulder muscles to lift up. *Drishti* is the same as Position 5 (photo below).

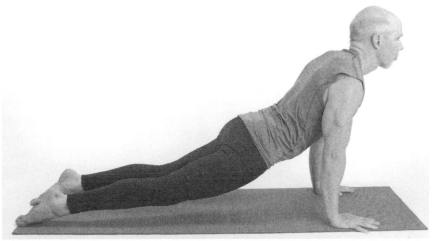

SUN SALUTATION POSITION 5, FACE UP DOG POSTURE, ADVANCED

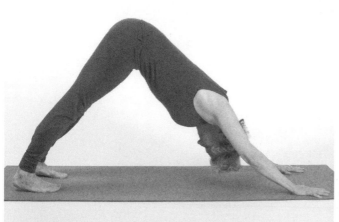

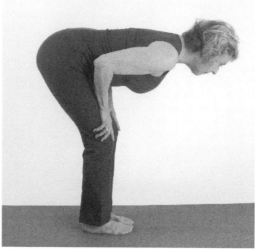

SUN SALUTATION POSITION 6, FACE DOWN DOG POSTURE

SUN SALUTATION POSITION 7

POSITION 6

Exhale as you change the position of your feet again, so the toes are turned back under.

Push up and back into an upside-down V-position or what is called Face Down Dog Posture.

Look back between your legs to a point behind you. This is your *drishti*.

Let your head and neck relax. Once you come into this position you are going to hold this posture for five complete controlled *ujjayi* breaths (one complete breath equals one inhalation and one exhalation).

POSITION 7

This is the same posture as Position 3 that you did on the way down.

Inhale as you step or hop your feet back to your hands. Bend your knees slightly (don't jump into a squat — it's hard on the knees!). Place your hands on your knees (or the floor) and arch and extend the back. *Drishti* is looking up.

Position 6 is an awesome place to hang out. It stretches the hamstrings, the calves, the back, the tendons in your ankles and feet, and strengthens the arms and shoulders. Push down on your heels. Pull up on the belly. Be mindful not to let your elbows lock out or hyperextend, which means to press inward. If this is your tendency, soften your elbows slightly and let them curve out the tiniest bit like parenthesis.

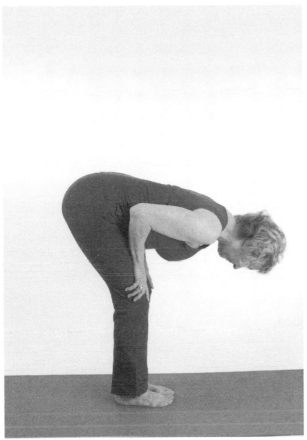

SUN SALUTATION POSITION 8

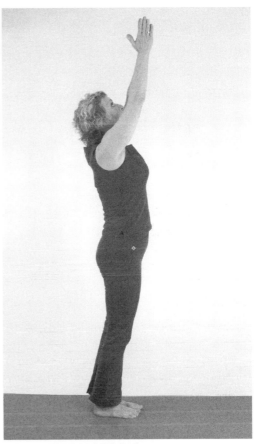

SUN SALUTATION POSITION 9

POSITION 8

This is the same pose as Position 2 that you did on the way down.

Exhale as you round the back slightly and tuck the nose toward the chest, keeping your hands on your knees (or on the floor). *Drishti* is looking down.

POSITION 9

This is the same as Position 1.

Inhale as you come all the way back up to standing, arms parallel over your head or palms touching. *Drishti* is gazing up at thumbs or looking straight out in front of you. Remember to hold your belly in, level the pelvis, and tuck in the tailbone.

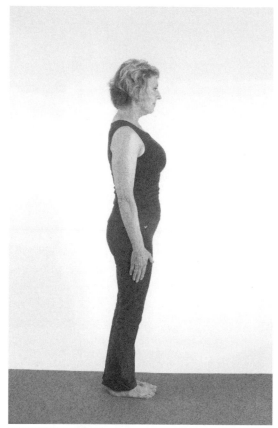

MOUNTAIN POSTURE

After completing Sun Salutation Position 9, exhale, bring your arms back down to your sides, returning to the way you began in Mountain Posture (or Attention Position).

Stand with your feet together, spine straight, natural curves in place (photo left). Make sure your belly is pulled in, pelvis level, thighs engaged (or contracted, which pulls up the knee caps), and visualize your shoulder blades melting down your back. Keep your gaze steady.

Be careful not to hyperextend the knees; you can soften the knees slightly and still contract the thighs. Breathe. This completes one full Sun Salutation. Repeat the sequence 3 times. Work up to 5 repetitions as you become stronger.

If you have been practicing the Sun Salutations for awhile now, learned the movements and feel comfortable flowing through them, then they will be followed directly by the Standing Postures in the next chapter. But when starting out, only do this much. This will only take about 5 minutes, so no one can say they don't have the time for this. Close your mouth and just do it.

When you have finished your Sun Salutations, lie down on your mat, on your back, and bring your knees up to your chest. Give yourself a hug and roll your knees from one side to the other, while keeping your shoulders on the ground. This is Lying Down Spinal Twist Posture (photo left).

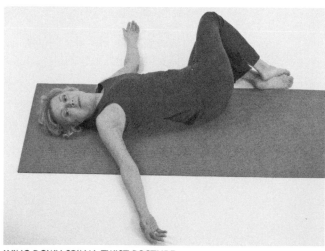

LYING DOWN SPINAL TWIST POSTURE

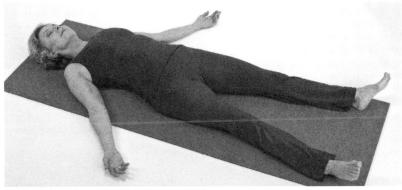

RELAXATION POSTURE

Then return your knees to the center and stretch your legs out full-length along your mat. Place your feet hip-width apart, then allow them to just fall open to the sides.

Check to make sure your head is level and your chin isn't jutting up toward the ceiling. Take your arms slightly out from your sides and turn the palms so they are facing up. Close your eyes. This is called Relaxation Posture (photo above).

See if you can keep your attention on your breathing. Let the breath become quieter and quieter, softer and softer, slower and slower, dropping the *ujjayi* breathing and returning to natural breath. Stay here as you cool down and drop into relaxation — for at least 5 minutes and preferably 10.

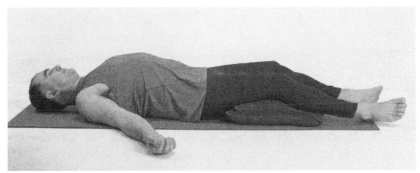

SUPPORTED RELAXATION POSTURE

Remember, if your back didn't hurt before you began your yoga practice, it shouldn't hurt after your yoga practice. If it does, you are doing something wrong. If you have chronic lower-back soreness or tightness, this practice should help to loosen the tight muscles and heal any injuries or alleviate misalignment. However, if you experience any tightness or discomfort in your back when you come into Relaxation Posture, it may be helpful to place a fairly sturdy pillow or bolster or folded-up blanket under your knees.

EXERCISE CHART - SUN SALUTATION

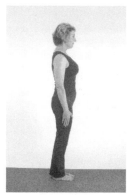

MOUNTAIN POSTURE

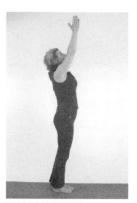

SUN SALUTATION
POSITION 1

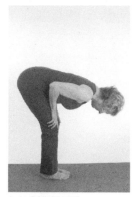

SUN SALUTATION
POSITION 2

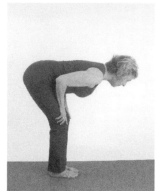

SUN SALUTATION
POSITION 3

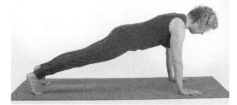

SUN SALUTATION POSITION 4, PLANK POSTURE

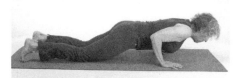

SUN SALUTATION POSITION 4

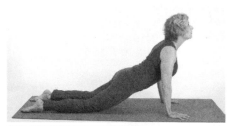

SUN SALUTATION, POSITION 5

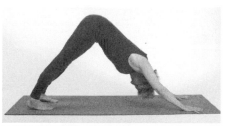

SUN SALUTATION POSITION 6

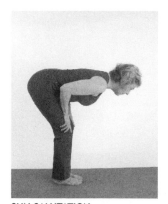

SUN SALUTATION
POSITION 7

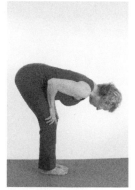

SUN SALUTATION
POSITION 8

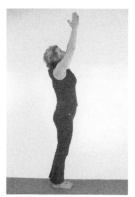

SUN SALUTATION
POSITION 9

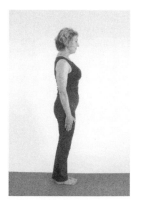

MOUNTAIN POSTURE

EXERCISE CHART - RELAXATION POSTURES

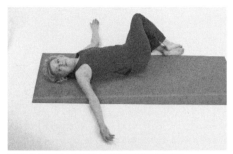

LYING DOWN SPINAL TWIST POSTURE

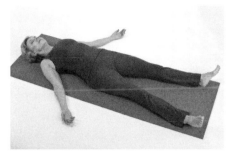

RELAXATION POSTURE

STRETCHING AND STRENGTHENING

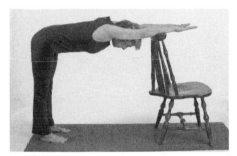

CHAIR HANG

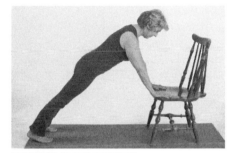

MODIFIED PLANK POSTURE

These are two great posture variations that you can do to work on your shoulders and arms. Chair Hang will help you to open up and relieve tightness in your shoulders. Doing mini-push-ups in Modified Plank Posture will build strength in your arms.

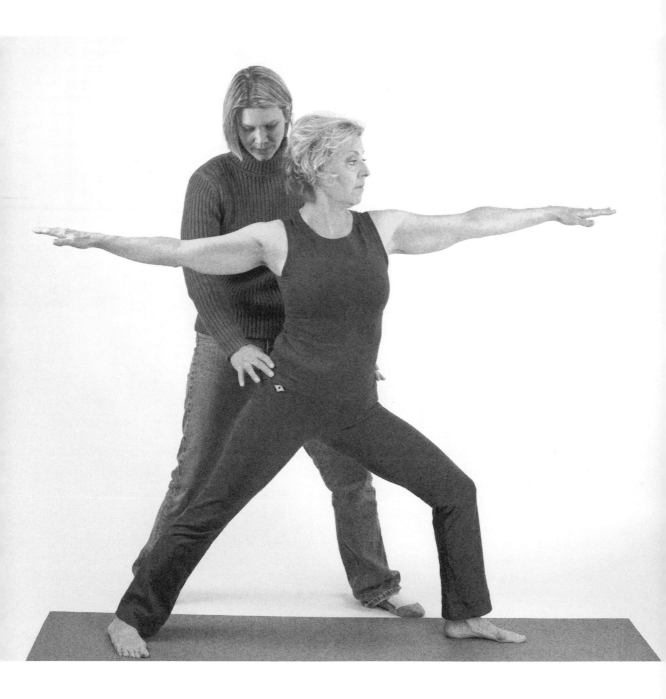

Chapter 4 POWER AND BALANCE

Getting Your Attention in Present Time

Keep in mind, you are developing a practice. This is a discipline that will take time to master. You can take it as far or near as you like. But it is still designed as a discipline, which makes it a little different from just another form of exercise. If you are in a hurry, this is not for you. This practice will not, as I like to say, take you from stupid to smart, tight to flexible, fat to fit, or injured to repaired, in twenty-one days or less.

Maybe all you will ever do is the Sun Salutation, and that will fix your problems or fill the expectations you have of yoga. That's fine. But no matter how much of the *asana* training you ever do, if you are really interested in the methodology or study of yoga, you should probably take a minute to understand how the word "practice" is defined in classical yoga.

The Yoga Sutra, as we've talked about previously, is the classical text on traditional yoga. Originally composed in Sanskrit, the secret messages of yoga were only available to those who could read the language — the Brahmin priests and Sanskrit scholars. That left the rest of us poor unenlightened souls in the dark. Today, however, we have lots of translations available. In Swami Satchidananda's translation, published in 1978, the definition of *abhyasa*, or "practice" is given in Book 1, Sutra 13, and defined as "effort towards steadiness of mind." This was captivating to me when I first discovered it about twenty years ago. It didn't say anything about stretching or building a yoga butt. It said, "Pay attention to whatever it is you are doing." That's what is meant by *practice* in yoga — if you aren't making an effort to get your attention in present time, for example, while you are doing your *asana* practice then it isn't really *practice*, it's just exercise. There's nothing wrong with exercise — it just isn't yoga.

But looking a little further, wouldn't that mean, if practice is defined as "effort towards steadiness of mind," that yoga practice isn't just about *asana* but it is something that can be done 24/7? Gee, you may think, all I wanted was to stretch out my hamstrings and suddenly I realize that yoga is training me in ways I didn't even realize when I started this simple activity called *asana*! Yoga teaches us that if we can learn to pay attention while we are doing the Sun Salutation, then maybe we can learn to pay attention while we are taking a shower, walking the dog, talking with our boss, or standing in line at the bank. It is about mindfulness. You may ask, "So why would we want to focus just on what we happen to be doing at the moment? Don't we want to do eighty-seven things at once? Isn't that the way of the twenty-first century? Don't people pride themselves on multi-tasking?"

A slightly more esoteric version of *abhyasa* (practice), from the translation by Mukunda Stiles reads, "The constant struggle to stay firmly rooted in the stable state of the True Self." That translation is a little more obscure, but I think we can still figure it out. Who in the world is the True Self? Well, after all the smoke and mirrors clear, isn't that what we really want to know? I mean, why do we even want to do yoga? Just to get flexible? Relaxed? Maybe, but it's a lot of work. Wouldn't it be easier to just watch TV or read a mystery novel? Deep down, maybe subconsciously, I think we also want to be centered, grounded, more conscious, more awake, and more in touch with our innermost being. Forget all the pseudo-sacred hocus-pocus found in today's world of post-traditional spiritual values. Plain and simple, what we want to know is, Who am I really? Yoga has an answer, but it's buried in the practice — your practice.

The *Sutra* goes on to tell us, importantly, not only what practice is, but how to get it firmly grounded. To be worth a hoot, practice needs to be three things — it must be done for a *dirga kala* (long time), *nairantarya* (without a break), and with *satkara* (earnestness). Well, that about covers it, wouldn't you

say? Bummer — no way around commitment it seems! So you see what I mean when I say, "This is a discipline." The methodology was conceived about 2200 years ago to help human beings evolve — physically, mentally, and spiritually. How far anyone wanted to go was totally up to them. But the bottom line was that to tap into the heavy-duty benefits of the program, a person actually needed to commit (imagine, they were talking about "commitment" 2200 years ago!) to actually doing it — consistently and for an extended period of time (read "for life!").

THE MINDFULNESS TOOLS

This practice gives us three basic tools for use in *asana* to help us get started in the work of learning to pay attention. In the last chapter we learned about two of them — *ujjayi* breathing and *drishti* (the gazing point). You may be inclined to just slide over them. But they aren't throwaway lines. They are integral, essential, and critical to doing the work properly. The *ujjayi* breathing technique just has to be learned correctly. There is no way around it. Without it, you just aren't doing yoga. So spend time learning it and practicing it — and not just when you are doing *asana*, but all the time. You may "learn" the *ujjayi* technique fairly quickly (hopefully you will) and you will think you've "got it." But over the years as you practice, the breath evolves, changing constantly, becoming more and more and more refined and controlled, just as the activity of the mind will become more conscious and controlled.

Learning to use *drishti* is a bit more difficult at first. The mind — in most cases — simply does not want to be restricted in its range of entertainment, and since most of our entertainment comes to us through our senses, to limit one of them — the sense of sight — is irritating to us. So you will probably find it difficult, if not annoying, to try and hold your gaze steady in the postures. At this point, it is good to remember the definition of practice — the effort towards steadiness of mind. If you are jumping around with your eyes, triggering this thought and that, then you are *not* making an effort to keep your mind steady. All this takes time. You will see how it works as you make your way through the book.

So before you rush on to more postures and more information, let yourself practice the less tangible aspects of the training — *drishti* and *ujjayi*. Instead of just trying to look good in the postures, see if you can actually put some effort into focusing on the breathing and holding your gaze steady.

PREPARING FOR THE STANDING POSTURES

This chapter will introduce you to what are called Standing *Asanas* or Postures. I have included ten postures in this section of the practice. If you are just starting out with a yoga practice, these postures should be learned one at a time, adding maybe one or two to your workout every couple of days. If you have been practicing yoga for some time and are knowledgeable about alignment, then you can work through the sequence at a somewhat faster pace. When I first learned the yoga practice (that this sequence is based upon) from my teacher, Norman Allen, I just did Sun Salutations for the first week, slowly increasing the number of repetitions. By the end of the second week I was doing probably about six repetitions, and then adding one or two Standing Postures. Every day I went to practice, I would repeat what I did the day before, adding a bit more to the routine every few days or weeks, slowly building strength and concentration.

After you have completed your last Sun Salutation, and stepped back to the top of your mat into Mountain Posture, you will begin the first Standing Posture. Check your feet, make sure they are aligned: toes touching, or feet parallel, grounded, even and balanced between *pronation* (rolling in) and *supination* (rolling out). If you have flat feet or collapsed arches, especially pay attention to pressing a bit more on the outside of your feet, being mindful to consciously "lift" your arches.

GENERAL GUIDELINES FOR ALL POSTURES

Now that we have arrived at this point, and you have done a little work, you will be better able to understand some general guidelines that will help you to refine your practice. Once learned, the postures are meant to be done sequentially, flowing from one to the next, from one side to the other, using the breath to move the body in and out of the postures. Here are some additional tips that will help you.

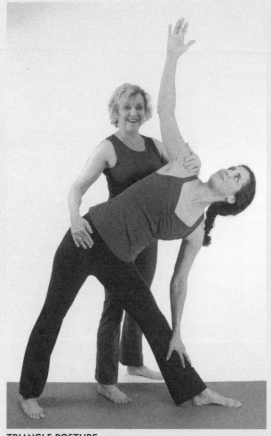

TRIANGLE POSTURE

- Balance the weight evenly on both feet for all the Standing Postures (the postures in chapter 4).

- Don't hold your breath, keep it flowing. Sixty or 70 percent of your effort, as you go along, is going to be in keeping the breathing "pump" going strongly — not through straining, but through clear focus.

- You will be moving up and down into the postures. Every movement is accompanied by an inhalation or an exhalation. Listen to you breath and practice paying attention to it. Try to coordinate the duration of a connecting movement with the duration of the breath — generally you will be exhaling going into a posture and inhaling coming out.

- Don't be sloppy. Sloppy doesn't do anything. Yoga isn't yoga if it's sloppy. Pay attention to the correct alignment of the posture. All the postures require strength, which means some muscles are working! Don't just flop into a posture and hang out. Find your strength.

- Pay attention to your head and neck — don't let them hang in the postures. The head is an extension of the spine and should be held in alignment with the spine in the postures.

- Especially pay attention to the alignment of the feet. If the directions say turn the right foot out 90 degrees — make sure it's 90 degrees and not 89. It makes a difference. Don't just read this and forget about it. Make a sign and hang it up where you will be practicing that says "FEET!!!"

- If anything you do hurts, you are doing it wrong. Back off whatever you are doing until it stops hurting. Or skip it altogether.

- Once you have "found" your posture, settle in and try not to fidget. See if you can come to stillness as you take your 5 breaths. Keep the gaze steady as well.

- Be aware of the balance between the "hard" energy of the muscles that are contracting in any posture, and the "soft" energy of the muscles that are relaxed or stretching. Often you will find that you are going a bit over the balance point toward one end of the spectrum or the other. Too much contraction results in straining and can lead to injury. Too much relaxation results in "sleeping" and can lead to not much of anything in terms of change or transformation.

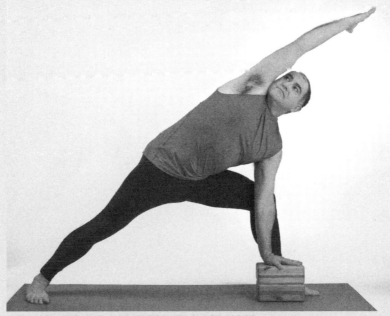

EXTENDED SIDE ANGLE POSTURE WITH BLOCK ASSIST

THE STANDING POSTURES

TRIANGLE POSTURE

1. *Inhale*, from the top of your mat, turn to your right and step your feet 3 feet apart. Make your feet parallel and then turn your right foot out 90 degrees and your left foot in 45 degrees. Lift your arms, parallel to the floor. Tighten the right thigh muscle.

NOTE: Consciously holding the quadriceps (thigh muscles) in static contraction on the forward leg is vitally important to the correct practice of the posture. This helps to protect the hamstrings (muscles at the back of the thigh), maintain heat, support the torso, and hold the knee in correct alignment. This is tricky. It doesn't happen automatically — you have to do it mindfully, and if you are tight, you will have a difficult time because all your attention will be focused on how tight you are. Practice engaging and holding this contraction before you go into the posture. You can tell you are doing it correctly because your kneecap will lift up.

2. *Exhale*, bend to the right, taking hold of your shin or ankle or whatever you can reach. Turn your head and look up at your left hand. This is the *drishti*. Hold for 5 breaths. Keep your arms and shoulders aligned in a vertical plane as best you can. If you can, grab your big toe with your first two fingers for a more advanced posture but don't bend your knee. After your last exhalation,

3. *Inhale* and come up out of the posture, reverse your feet — precisely — and

4. *Exhale* and descend into the posture on the other side (photo below). *Drishti* is up at the right hand. Hold for 5 breaths. After your 5th exhalation, then

5. *Inhale*, move up out of the posture, turn both feet facing forward, so they are parallel, and

6. *Exhale*, step back to the top of your mat, feet together. Go directly to the next posture.

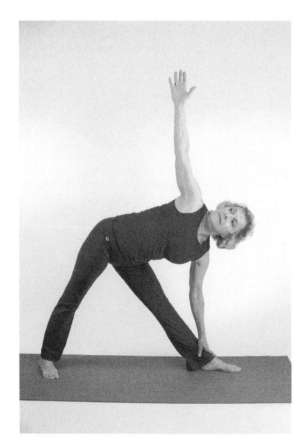

TRIANGLE POSTURE

DOING THE WORK

When I was younger I was more interested in how proficient I was at the postures and how my muscles were responding. Now I'm more focused on how I'm using my *prana* (energy) and where my attention is going. What happens to the breath when a posture is easy? Difficult? What about the mind? Where is your attention going, and consequently, your energy? What are the ways in which you are wasting energy? What thoughts are distracting you?

If you are just starting out with yoga, or even if you have been doing *asana* practice for some time, it's important for you to begin to develop your ability to notice when you are distracted and what it is that has distracted you. If your objective is to keep your mind on your breathing, and all of a sudden you are thinking about selling your house and moving to Colorado, well, you've been distracted. And it may take a few moments before you even realize it. But once you become conscious of the fact that you aren't here any longer, but off in the Rocky Mountains somewhere, it is important that you bring your attention back to the present moment. Often the mind doesn't want to let go of whatever it is that it is thinking about — it's delicious, it's tantalizing, it's challenging, it's stimulating. All the more important to let it go and come back to the breath! Perhaps, you never made an effort to check your thoughts before and keep your attention present. But this is an essential skill to develop early on in your yoga practice, as it will prepare your body and mind for the more subtle practices that follow in later chapters. I call it "doing the work."

Spend enough time with the Standing Postures to learn the sequence by heart. Do it three or four times a week for three or four weeks or longer. No rush. Take your time. Develop mindfulness.

EXTENDED SIDE ANGLE POSTURE

1. *Inhale* and step to the right, taking your feet 5 feet apart, or as far as you can, this time. Turn the right foot out 90 degrees and the left foot in 45 degrees. Raise the arms and

2. *Exhale*, bend your right knee to a 90-degree angle, so the knee is directly over the ankle, and take your right elbow to rest on your right thigh. Reach your left arm out over your head and ear. Put your strength into it all the way to the finger tips. If you can't sink into your hips that far, use a block or a phone book to support you (photo below, right).

3. Keep your head in alignment with the spine. Do not throw the head back to look up at the hand, which is a common mistake. Keep the chin tucked into the armpit. Just look up with your eyes! Come to still-ness. *Drishti* is at the left hand. Hold for 5 breaths. After your last exhalation,

4. *Inhale*, move up and out of the position, reverse your feet — exactly, and

5. *Exhale*, descend into the posture on the other side (photo below, left). *Drishti* is now at the right hand. Remember to keep your chin tucked. Hold for 5 breaths. After your 5th exhalation, you are going to go directly into the next posture.

TWISTED SIDE ANGLE POSTURE

1. *Inhale*, reverse your feet once again, going back to where you started for Extended Side Angle, right foot turned out, left foot turned in.

2. *Exhale*, bend your knee and twist your

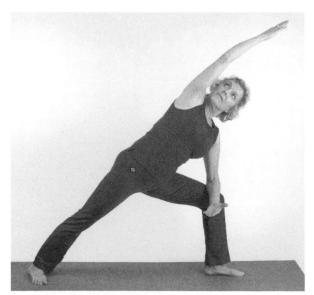

EXTENDED SIDE ANGLE POSTURE

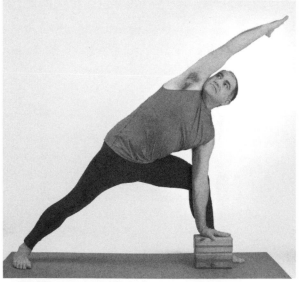

EXTENDED SIDE ANGLE POSTURE WITH BLOCK ASSIST

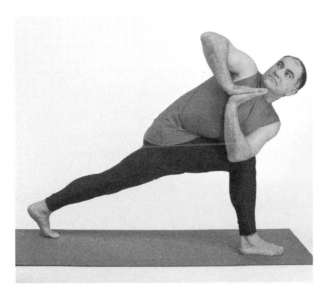

TWISTED SIDE ANGLE POSTURE

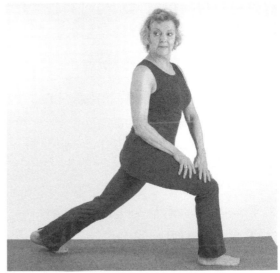

TWISTED SIDE ANGLE POSTURE, MODIFIED

torso, now taking your left elbow or back of your left arm (the triceps) to your right thigh. Bring your palms together and push them into one another. Try to "sink" into the posture, dropping your hips. Don't fidget. *Drishti* is out of the right corners of your eyes, looking back. Hold for 5 breaths. If you can't sink into your hips quite that far, then just keep your torso upright and twist (photo above, right). After your 5th exhalation,

3. *Inhale* and move up out of the posture,

reverse your feet — precisely — and

4. *Exhale* and descend into the posture on the other side. Hold for 5 breaths. After your 5th exhalation, then

5. *Inhale*, move up out of the posture, square yourself off (making feet parallel again) and

6 *Exhale*, step back to the top of your mat. Feet together. Go directly to the next posture.

Make an effort to twist as far around as you can, first trying to move the back of the left arm, then the left shoulder as close as possible to (or even beyond) the right knee. Use your arms to give you leverage to work on the twist and open the right shoulder back. Be careful not to push so hard that you shove your knee out of alignment. You will need to push back with your knee against your arm to find balance. If it is easier, you can lift the heel of the back foot, turning it out and coming up on your toes. Balance is a little trickier, but the twist is easier. Keep in mind that most of the twist is happening in the thoracic (middle) portion of the spine. This should not strain your lower back.

EXPANDED LEG STRETCH WITH ARMS OVERHEAD POSTURE

1. *Inhale* and step to the right, taking your feet 5 feet apart again, as in the last posture. This time you will keep the feet parallel. Check and make sure they are. They probably aren't. Lift your arms out to the sides, parallel to the floor. Tighten your thighs — and keep them that way!

2. *Exhale*, interlace your hands behind your back. If you have tight pectoralis (front of shoulders) muscles, this may be difficult. Do what you can.

3. *Inhale*, straighten your arms. Put your strength into it. Press the wrists together. Stretch back a little, opening the chest and heart center. Keep the tailbone dropped and the pelvis level (photo below, left).

4. *Exhale*, bend forward, tipping the pelvis forward and lifting the tailbone, taking your hands over your head. Keep thighs contracted! Keep the head in line with the spine. (photo below, right and opposite page, left). The tendency as you bend

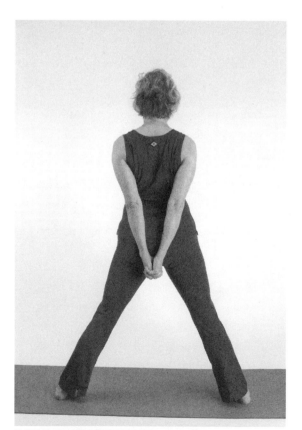

EXPANDED LEG STRETCH POSTURE, BACK

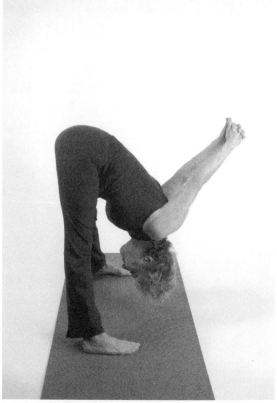

EXPANDED LEG STRETCH POSTURE, SIDE

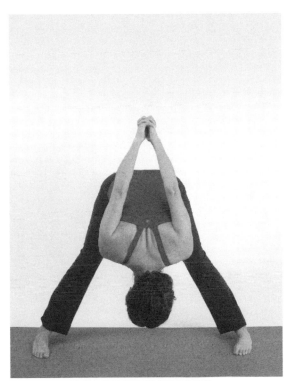

EXPANDED LEG STRETCH POSTURE, FRONT

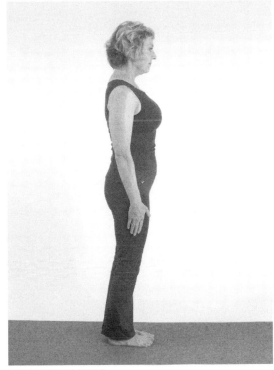

MOUNTAIN POSTURE

forward will be to let the wrists come apart so you can take the arms a little farther overhead. This is a little risky as it can lead to overstretching or hyperextending the elbows. *Drishti* is out past the end of your nose. Take 5 breaths. After your 5th exhalation,

5. *Inhale*, look up, and come up halfway.

6. *Exhale* in place.

7. *Inhale*, come up the rest of the way to standing. Squeeze the shoulder blades together and keep pelvis tucked under.

8. *Exhale*, release the posture and step back to Mountain Posture at the top of your mat.

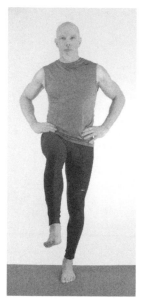

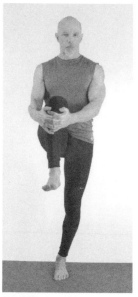

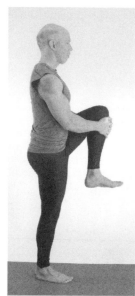

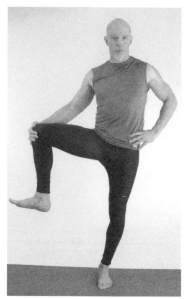

STANDING KNEE TO CHEST
POSTURE A

STANDING KNEE TO CHEST
POSTURE B

STANDING KNEE TO CHEST
POSTURE B

STANDING KNEE TO CHEST
POSTURE C

STANDING KNEE TO CHEST
POSTURE A, B, AND C

Before you begin these postures, find a *drishti* first — straight out in front of you. Lock your eyes on that point and don't let them drift. This is critical for balance, as the better your concentration, the better your balance. Put your strength into this posture. Contract the thighs, pull up through the torso, pull the belly in, and roll the shoulders back.

1. *Inhale*, starting with feet together. Lift the right leg and bend the knee, raising it as high as you can.

2. *Exhale*, lift the toes (dorsiflex the foot) and keep the shin perpendicular to the floor, with the foot directly under the knee. Place your hands on your hips. This is Posture A. Take 5 breaths. Remember, *drishti* is straight out in front

of you. After your 5th exhalation,

3. *Inhale*, reach your arms towards your knee and grab hold of the knee, without shifting your gaze,

4. *Exhale*, pull the knee into the chest for Posture B. Use your arms to pull, engaging the bicep muscles. Lift the chest. Stand tall. The foot should remain directly under the knee and the shin perpendicular to the floor. *Drishti* is the same as Posture A. Take 5 breaths. After your 5th exhalation,

5. *Inhale*, then exhale and open the leg to the right side for Posture C. *Drishti* stays the same. Take 5 breaths. After your 5th exhalation,

6. *Inhale* and move the leg back to the front.

7. *Exhale*, pull knee to chest once more.

8. *Inhale* and hold. Exhale, release posture, returning to Mountain Posture, with feet together, standing at "attention." Repeat instructions for left side. Then, go directly to the next posture.

STANDING HALF LOTUS POSTURE

1. *Inhale*, starting with feet together, lift the right foot, grasping the ankle with both hands raising it as high as you can, and

2. *Exhale*, pulling the foot in toward the left hip bone. Keep the knee level or angled up slightly. Do not push down the knee (see Note). Engage the arm muscles, using your arm strength to pull the heel in and up toward the left half of your belly (abdomen) (top photo). If you are able, take the right arm around behind you and grab hold of the left forearm (photo, right). *Drishti* is straight out in front of you. Take 5 breaths. After your last exhalation, inhale, then exhale, release the posture.

3. Repeat instructions for the left side. Return to Mountain Posture.

NOTE: For some reason people don't want to keep their knee up in this posture, even if I am standing in front of them explaining it. Keeping the knee high is a much less stressful position for the knee. If your knee feels at all tweaky while you are doing this, lift, lift, lift it higher until it stops feeling funny and *try to point it forward, as opposed to out to the side.* This facilitates stretching out the

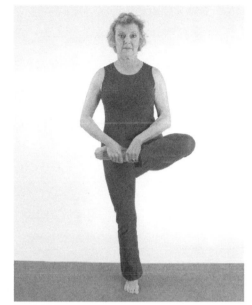

STANDING HALF LOTUS POSTURE

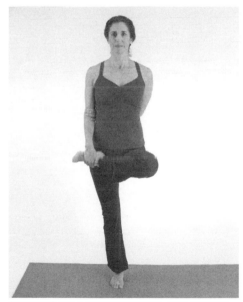

STANDING HALF LOTUS POSTURE, ARM BEHIND

gluteus medius (a muscle in your butt that helps to abduct, or open the legs out to the sides) and makes sitting cross legged easier. It also further protects the knee.

VINYASA TO FIERCE POSTURE

Instead of just going into Fierce Posture directly from Mountain Posture, we are going to move through what in yoga has come to be colloquially referred to as *vinyasa*. Figuratively, it means flowing movement or series of movements that takes you from one posture to another. Literally, it means to set down, or to place carefully. So the opening *vinyasa* for this posture corresponds to the first 6 movements of the Sun Salutation and the following 7 instructions will review it for you.

VINYASA SEQUENCE

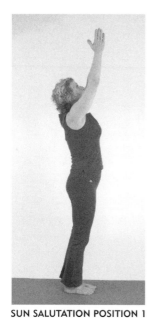

SUN SALUTATION POSITION 1

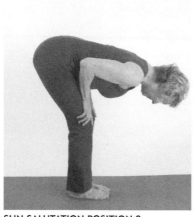

SUN SALUTATION POSITION 2

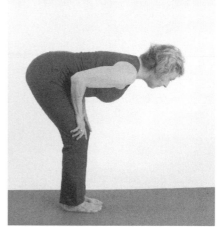

SUN SALUTATION POSITION 3

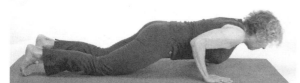

SUN SALUTATION POSITION 4

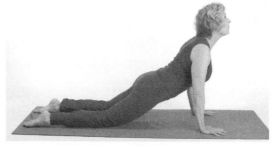

SUN SALUTATION POSITION 5, FACE UP DOG POSTURE

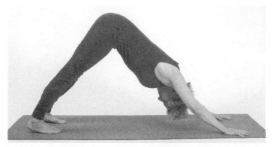

SUN SALUTATION POSITION 6, FACE DOWN DOG POSTURE

1. *Inhale*, take the arms up overhead, look up. (Sun Salutation Position 1)

2. *Exhale*, take the hands to the knees, look down and back toward the navel. (Sun Salutation Position 2)

3. *Inhale*, hands stay on knees, look up. (Sun Salutation Position 3)

4. *Exhale*, take your hands to the floor and walk or jump the legs back and come into the push-up position. (Sun Salutation Position 4)

5. *Inhale*, come into Face Up Dog Posture (Sun Salutation Position 5), then

6. *Exhale*, come into Face Down Dog Posture (Sun Salutation Position 6), then

7. *Inhale*, walk or jump the feet up to the hands.

FIERCE POSTURE

1. *Exhale*, bend the knees, raise the torso, and bring the arms over the head, palms pressing together if possible. Lean forward slightly. Sink as deeply as you comfortably can and raise the arms as high as you can. *Drishti* is up at your hands. (If this is uncomfortable for your neck, just look straight ahead.) Take 5 breaths.

After your 5th exhalation, you will again put in a couple of movements from the Sun Salutation sequence to take you into the last two Standing Postures:

2. *Inhale*, take your hands to your knees (or to the floor) and look up (Sun Salutation Position 3).

3. *Exhale*, hands to the floor and walk or jump back to your push-up position (Sun Salutation Position 4).

4. *Inhale*, come into Face Up Dog Posture (Sun Salutation Position 5), then

5. *Exhale*, come into Face Down Dog Posture (Sun Salutation Position 6). Go directly into the next posture.

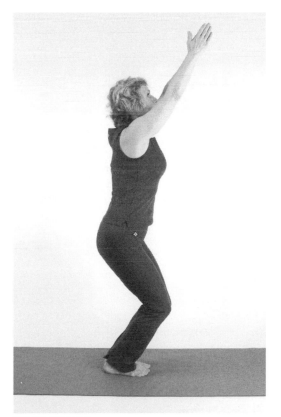

FIERCE POSTURE

WARRIOR I POSTURE

1. *Inhale*, from Face Down Dog Posture, step the right foot all the way up to a point between your hands, or as close as you can get, and turn the left heel in toward the midline of your body. Keep the left foot flat on the floor and press on the outside edge of the foot. The left foot should now be angled in about 45 degrees and anchored to the floor.

2. *Exhale*, raise the arms up overhead, palms touching if possible. Otherwise, just make the arms parallel. *Drishti* is up at your hands or straight in front of you. Settle in. Take 5 breaths.

3. *Inhale*, straighten the right leg and reverse your feet, so that you have turned completely around 180 degrees.

4. *Exhale*, bend the left knee over the left ankle and repeat the posture on the left side. Go directly into the next posture.

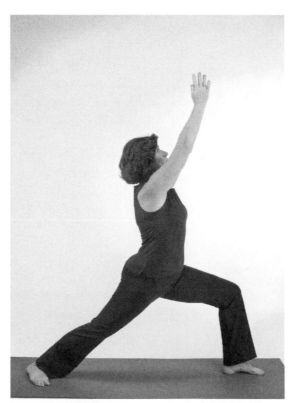

WARRIOR I POSTURE

Most of the problems in this posture come as a result of tight hips and tight shoulders, which many of us have. This tightness is not uncommon in athletes of almost all varieties. If your hips are tight, then it is going to be tough to step your foot all the way up to your hands from Face Down Dog Posture as you won't have the range of motion in your hips. In this case, you'll need to shorten the stance, which is fine (photo below, left). Just step up as far as you can, making sure that the heel of the front foot is in a line with the heel of the back foot. Just as in the Sun Salutation, tight shoulders will prevent you from taking your arms directly overhead. If you don't have the range of motion you need, just take your arms as high as you can without leaning back, which will stress the lower back. Keep the tailbone dropped, the ribcage tucked, and the belly pulled in, just as in Mountain Posture. It's really important to pay attention to alignment on all fronts in this posture — the feet, hips, back, knees, shoulders, neck, and head. A really great way to get a "sense" of the posture, both to facilitate the stretch in the back leg and to develop the strength you need to actually do the posture in the thigh of your front leg, is to use a chair to support your front leg (photo below, right).

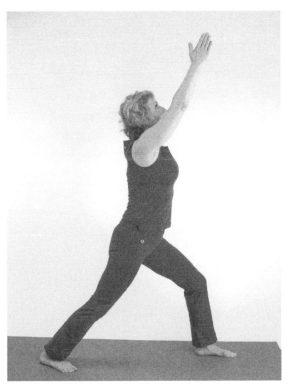

WARRIOR I POSTURE, SHORTER STANCE

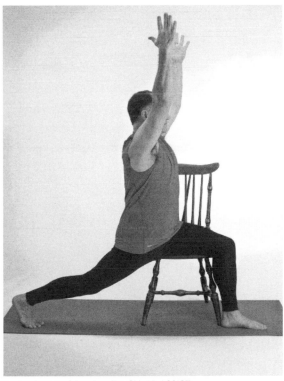

WARRIOR I POSTURE WITH CHAIR ASSIST

WARRIOR II POSTURE

1. *Inhale*, swing the arms down and out, so they are parallel to the floor and in line with your legs.

2. *Exhale*, shift torso and hips to the right. Torso will turn 90 degrees, but how far the hips can shift will depend on their relative tightness or flexibility. Your arms, torso, and hips are now in line with the plane of the legs. Be careful not to let your left knee cave in. Keep it centered over the ankle. Drop (or tuck) the tailbone and pull the belly in. Keep the pelvis level. You are still on your left side, so the *drishti* is out at the tips of your left fingers. Take 5 breaths. After your 5th exhalation,

3. *Inhale*, straighten the left leg, reverse your feet, and

4. *Exhale*, bend the right knee over the right ankle and repeat Warrior II to the right side. *Drishti* is at your right fingertips. Hold for 5 breaths. After your 5th exhalation, go into the following vinyasa sequence.

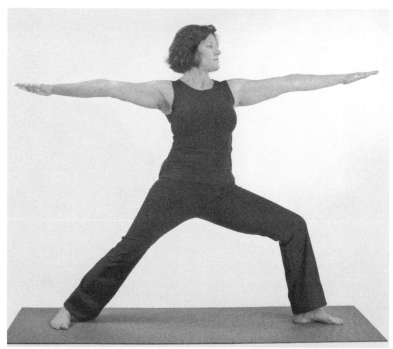

WARRIOR II POSTURE

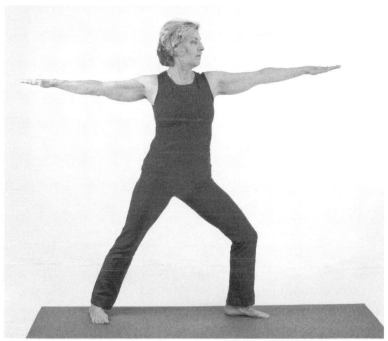

WARRIOR II POSTURE, SHORTER STANCE

5. *Inhale*, take your hands to the floor along-side your right foot, then

6. *Exhale*, walk or jump back into your push-up position.

7. *Inhale*, come into Face Up Dog Posture, then

8. *Exhale*, come into Face Down Dog Posture.

9. *Inhale*, hop your feet up towards your hands, bend your knees, cross your ankles, and

10. *Exhale*, sit down. Go directly to the first Seated Posture, or, if you are ending your practice here, go directly into Relaxation Posture (page 47).

Well, that's it for the Standing Postures. It may seem easy, or it may seem hard. If you are tight from years of training, sports, life, kids, injuries, abuse, etc., this is going to be a little laborious. In the beginning, you may find that attempting to learn the alignment and movements is a bit of a struggle, generally annoying, and plain uncomfortable. That's okay. I don't really care if you like it or not when you start — just do it!!! You can tell me after a few months of regular practice if it was of any value. Eventually, you need to enjoy it, or you won't keep doing it. But discomfort at one time or another is a part of life for everyone, and it generally passes. As you do more, this gets easier and the grunting and groaning diminishes.

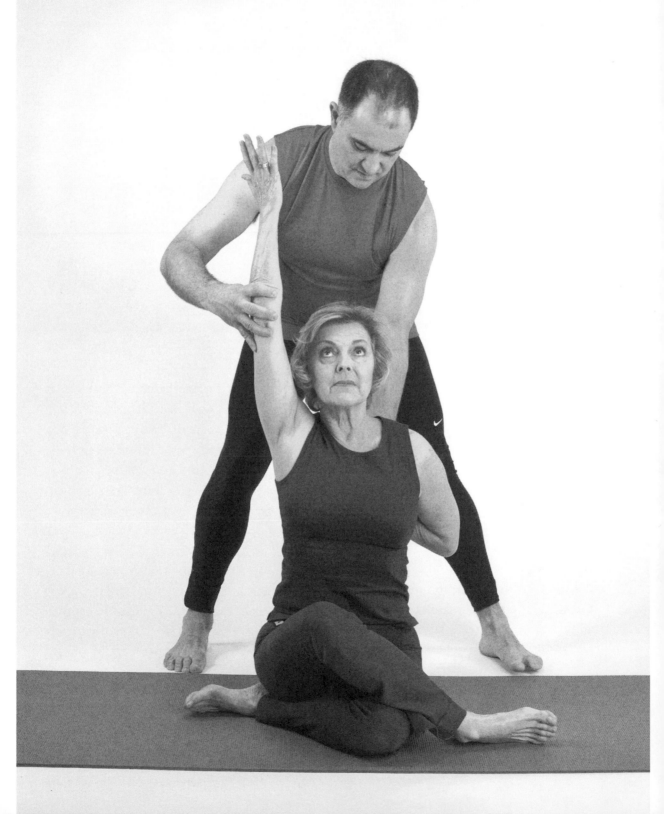

Chapter 5 **HARD & SOFT**

Finding Strength in Letting Go

One early February morning in 1976, when I was living in Fraser, Colorado, the "icebox of the nation," the temperature was 42 degrees below zero. That's 42 degrees below zero on the thermometer, not counting wind chill. The sun was blazing, the sky pristine, the day crystal clear, but it was friggin' cold! There wasn't much that happened on days like that except two things — getting cars started and thawing water pipes. Even with plug-in batteries for the cars and thermal wrap on the water pipes, there was a lot of cold that slipped through the cracks, so most everyone in town was pretty involved in generating some heat, one way or another.

At that time, I lived a couple miles out on the 4-Bar-4 Road. I had water, but my '64 Chevy Impala wouldn't start. Winter Park, the little town and the ski area, was just a few miles down route #40 to the east and was pretty much the hub of winter activity. I was due there in a few hours to teach my Yoga for Skiers class (of course), and was trying to figure out who I could call to come out and help me get my car started. I knew that just about everyone would be out dinking around with their cars or their pipes. Even the die-hard skiers generally skipped the slopes on mornings like this because they couldn't get there until they got their cars started!

The 4-Bar-4 Road was a dusty, dirt road and a bumpy, unpleasant ride in the summertime, but in the winter it was more like a luge track. It was a county road, so it did get plowed, but we had five-foot snow banks on either side (as we did almost every winter in Fraser Valley) and the road itself was beautifully snow-packed, so it was actually easier to drive on than it was in the summertime.

There were only a few folks who lived farther out than me, so waiting on the road for someone to pass was out of the question in terms of soliciting some help. Plus, the ones that did pass were going about fifty miles an hour, hurtling themselves towards the highway a few miles away. Asking anyone to stop, by flagging them down, was suicidal for us both. If they stopped abruptly, they would have gone soaring up one side of the road and then up the other, like a skate boarder at a park, or augured themselves in the snow-bank. If they stopped slowly, they would have taken the entire distance to the highway to come to a complete halt. It wasn't a good plan.

CHOPPING WOOD

I figured that before I set my mind to solving this car-won't-start problem, I'd get the wood-burning stove going. That was the first chore of the morning — every morning from mid-August, when the first snow appeared on the tops of the mountains, to late June, when the last snow melted, if you were lucky. My Alaskan husky Timber (who was part Siberian, part Samoyed, and part coyote) and I went outside to chop some wood. The great thing about this kind of cold in Colorado is that it is bone dry. I just put on a long-sleeved t-shirt, a hat, and some mittens, and went out to split a few rounds for firewood. It sounds impressive, but it was easy. The wood — big, standing-dead rounds — was cold and dry. To picture a "round," imagine a cucumber, lying sideways on your cutting board. Now imagine cutting it into big fat slices. That's a "round." A whole tree is generally sliced into about eighteen- to twenty-four-inch-wide rounds with a chain saw and then the rounds can be chopped into smaller pieces for firewood.

You put the round up on a chopping block (that's just another fat round), tap in a wedge, and whale away at it with a sledgehammer. It takes amazing eye/hand coordination and pretty good concentration. If you aren't paying attention, you can miss hitting the wedge entirely, in which case you are generally left cussing and recovering from misplaced impact. But if you hit it straight on, this huge round of wood just shatters into about four or five nice little split wood pieces. It's an awesome feeling when you get it right. That morning

I got it right. I split a couple of rounds easily and was happy. What a gorgeous day. Timber was frolicking around like it was midsummer and we were just kind of *there*. I remember the moment really well. It didn't matter that the car didn't start. Life was breathtakingly beautiful in that moment. I was happy and grateful for the wood and the mittens and the shelter and the water and all of it. I loved it. The logs were light and dry so I carried in an armload. They burn really easily, so with a little paper and a few bits of kindling that I sliced off the split wood, in a few minutes — *whoosh* — I had a roaring fire. It was heaven on earth and my favorite way to start the mornings. I still build a fire every day, first thing from October to May, living here on the East End of Long Island. And I imagine that I will continue to do the same, most anywhere I might ever live.

Anyway, once I got the fire started, I called around to my friends, but no one was answering their phones. We didn't have answering machines and voice mail back then, just a lot of ringing phones. Everyone was out holding hair dryers to their batteries and pipes. I laughed when no one answered because I knew they were all outside, freezing their asses off, doing the same thing I'd been doing — trying to get their cars started!

SYNCHRONICITY IN ACTION

I didn't have a long enough extension cord to do the hair dryer thing, so I figured I'd just walk to the highway and get a ride to Winter Park from there. So I bundled up, walked to the highway, and caught a ride almost immediately with one of my yoga students, John Hubbard.

"Hey Beryl, car won't start eh?"

It didn't take him long to figure out what I was doing walking along Highway #40 when it was 42 degrees below zero.

"Are you going to yoga class?" he asked.

"Yeah," I said, "are you?"

"You bet. Are you working tonight?" John knew I was a waitress at the Swiss House a couple of nights a week.

"Yeah, if I can get to work."

"I'll take you home after class and help you get your car going."

Something about splitting the wood rounds had connected me to the moment, to the present. I felt connected to everyone, everywhere. It was a spectacular feeling. It was an experience of boundlessness. I was just connected to the Earth in the most appropriate and inexplicable way. Everything about that day seemed to flow effortlessly and spill forward in synchronicity. First, I got the ride with John, who was going to class. Perfect. And a ride home and help with getting my car started. More perfect. But on the way, a small event occurred that would influence my philosophical teachings for the next thirty-three years and most likely, will continue to do so forever. When I jumped into John's car, I noticed a small book on Zen Buddhism sitting on the front seat. While I was warming my feet on the heater, I picked up the book and opened it at random,

to a place that had a Zen proverb listed at the top of the page. It caught my attention and I asked John about the book.

"Oh yeah, it's a great little book," he said. "I'm done with it. You can have it."

"Oh no, that's okay. I just like this little proverb here."

"No, really, you can have it."

"Really? Thanks."

The proverb was "*Only when you can be extremely pliable and soft, can you be extremely hard and strong.*" I don't remember the book; I just remember the proverb and for some reason it just exploded in my mind. It was like I had seen the light at the beginning of time. The heavens opened up and revealed the mysteries of the Universe. I suddenly understood that everything in life — and I mean everything — involved finding a balance between those two energies: hard and soft, hanging on and letting go, standing firm and surrendering, strengthening and stretching. I wrote it down and later that week, decided to call my various "enterprises" — from running wellness weeks, teaching yoga classes, and doing massage therapy to writing grants for humanities or sustainable-living projects — The Hard & The Soft whatever: The Hard & The Soft Yoga Center, The Hard & The Soft Growth Center, The Hard & The Soft Institute for the Humanities, The Hard & The Soft Massage Therapy, or whatever it was I was doing to support myself, which, in Colorado at the time, generally required a great deal of imagination and diversification.

FOLLOWING YOUR *DHARMA*

Buckminster Fuller has always been one of my mentors and I have always been a great admirer of his philosophy and world views. His book *Operating Manual for Spaceship Earth*, published in 1969, had a strong influence on the direction of my own personal beliefs. What really caught my attention in the most profound way was his idea that if you directed your work in a non-competitive, mindful, creative way that was supportive of the Universe, following your own *dharma* (a Sanskrit word that can mean one's "path" or "calling"), then the Universe would *literally* support you in all ways — physically, emotionally, and (although sometimes only in the nick of time) economically as well. The operative principle here was to be "non-competitive." Fuller teaches that you shouldn't try and do what someone else is doing. You have to find your own niche, your own path. This made perfect sense to me, in terms of what I already knew about *karma*, and it confirmed my worldview that if I pursued what in yoga is called "right action" to the best of my ability, then the Universe would take care of me. It's happened often in my life, like the time I adopted two Siberian huskies, Jesse and Gramfy, with the last $400 I had in my bank account, and then *the next day* I received a check in the mail for $400 from a friend and former student who said he was sending it for no particular reason other than he thought I might need it.

STRETCHING AND STRENGTHENING FOR ATHLETES

In 1980, I moved back to New York City and began teaching yoga classes through the New York Road Runners Club (NYRRC). I suggested using The Hard & The Soft Yoga as the title of the course but Fred Lebow, the founder and (at the time) president of the Club and the originator of the prestigious New York City Marathon, looked at me like I had just landed from Mars.

"Yoga?" he boomed. "The hard and the soft? Runners need to *stretch*! Why don't we call it *Stretching for Runners*?" Oh Gawd! I was horrified, but I didn't let it show, or at least not much. I wanted the job! Good Lord, if this kick-butt yoga *asana* practice called *ashtanga* that I had just discovered in New York was going to be offered as a class, I certainly didn't want it to fall into the category of (snore!) *stretching*. It wasn't just soft passive stretching, which is what most people tended to think yoga was all about. The *ashtanga* practice was both hard and soft, focusing equally on building strength as well as flexibility.

But I quickly realized we couldn't call it yoga. Believe it or not, the fitness market was not ready for anything remotely called "yoga" (much less "The Hard & The Soft Yoga"!) even in New York in 1980. I was primarily teaching athletes and the widespread perception about yoga at that time was that it was pretty "soft" and mostly for women. The attitude in the late '70s was that real men didn't do yoga, and that most women didn't do yoga either. So if I hoped to get anyone to my classes, then I needed to call those classes something other than "yoga." We settled on "Stretching and Strengthening for Athletes." That worked well for awhile and got the program off the ground, and then, after a few years, I decided to get a little more bold — and I re-titled the course "Yoga for Athletes!" and worked the idea of the "hard" and the "soft" into the descriptive copy.

As many of you know, over the years, "The Hard & The Soft" slowly became my "trademark," so to speak, and the foundation of my whole yoga practice and teaching philosophy. The brilliant idea, of finding the balance in yoga practice and eventually, in life, between the two opposing forces of the Universe, contraction and expansion, was philosophically intriguing to me and physiologically sound. I could actually physically teach people how to focus on the strength in this practice and balance it with the stretch, and they began to "get" the idea of "hard" and "soft." Since so many people still thought of yoga as something soft and relaxing, and an activity only engaged in by women, my idea was that it was important to let those same people know that this yoga was about both flexibility *and* strength and power! Ultimately, by 1985, this concept evolved into the name of my school, The Hard & The Soft Yoga Institute, which

began to offer yoga retreats and workshops and teacher training programs. But although it was a great name for a yoga school, and terrific as a philosophical concept, back in the dark ages of yoga in the West, the more esoteric message wasn't quite so clear and often left itself open to quite a bit of, let's say, misinterpretation.

Slowly, after teaching this "hard" and "soft" yoga practice to over one hundred thousand people in New York City between 1980 and 2002, the idea began to carry some weight. In 1990, when we were trying to update our yoga flyer that was mailed out monthly by the New York Road Runners Club to its 25,000 members, I came up with the name "power yoga." The name came to me early one morning in the middle of a meditation. Wow. Now there was a brand for a product! Everyone loved it and it helped to make clear that this yoga practice being offered at the NYRRC for athletes, was not just about "stretching." For me, the name was given by God. It described a powerful yoga system and was a name that Western minds could relate to. It also described a type of yoga that the fitness mentality of the '80s would be willing to at least try, and perhaps embrace as a viable alternative to their pounding '80s aerobic workouts. Well, a lot of people did try it and a lot a people got into yoga as a result of power yoga.

The name ran like wildfire through the media in the mid to late '90s, and when I tried to trademark the name, the Patent and Trademark Authority said that it wasn't "trademarkable," as it was a descriptive term. So "power yoga" — because it wasn't protected by a trademark — became anything anyone wanted it to be out there in the free marketplace, but my book, *Power Yoga*, became the gold standard for a "powerful" yoga practice and for a safe and effective way to learn a strong, *rajasic* (active) yoga practice. But the great thing about all this sharing of "power" was that it got many people doing yoga. Which teacher, which "power" yoga you ended up with depended on lots of factors: your location, your *karma*, your personality, your preferences, etc. As the yoga viewpoint tells us, "you get the teacher you are ready for." If you ended up with some yahoo teaching "power" yoga then hopefully it taught you discernment. None of it is a mistake. The entire phenomena paved the way for more and more people doing yoga, opening yoga studios, taking trips to India, and it also led to more yoga books, yoga clothes, yoga workshops, and all around more awareness about yoga!

BALANCING HARD AND SOFT

Five years after I adopted the whole exciting principle of the hard and the soft, I began my exploration of *The Yoga Sutra*, the ancient teachings of yoga collected by Patanjali, in which he lays out the actual eight-limbed path of classical yoga and then briefly explains each limb. Ironically, in the esoteric language of the 196 short but densely-packed-with-meaning verses that comprise the four chapters of *The Yoga Sutra*, Patanjali says almost nothing about *asana*. Apparently, he did not want to offend any of the existing *hatha* yoga schools by going into too much detail on any one particular system of yoga postures. But what he does emphasize about the practice of *asana* is the importance of finding the balance between *sthira*, Sanskrit for "steady, hard, focused," and *sukha*, Sanskrit for "easy, soft, comfortable." Aha! That's what I had thought, too — and not just about *asana*. Everything in life should be *sthira* and *sukha*! And I was soon to learn that Patanjali didn't just mean it to refer to *asana* either, but to the entire yoga journey through all eight limbs. I was wishing that Patanjali would just materialize and sit down for tea, so we could have a little chat about "hard" and "soft."

It seems to me that everything we do in life is about finding the balance between "hard" and "soft." No matter whether we are confronted with a difficult situation or relationship or making a decision on just about anything, we are always faced with the challenge of knowing just how much to "contract" or to stand our ground, and how much to "relax," or to let things pass. Do we settle at the restaurant for the lukewarm soup, or send it back? Is it okay the way it is, or should we ask for it to be really hot? We always wanted the corner office — do we fight for it, or does it really matter? What's the right thing to do? Our partner or spouse is most *definitely mistaken* about a particular matter. Do we push the issue or just let it go? Some things are easy to change or fix, others more difficult, and others impossible. Sometimes we are forced into action, other times we're forced into passivity, and still other times we get to choose the balance — how much *contraction* or how much *expansion* — we want to apply to a situation. And what is interesting about finding this balance, is that it must always be found in the present moment. Right here, right now. We can't really prepare by looking up in a book, for example, how much of each of these two fundamental energies of the Universe, needs to be applied in any given situation. But what I have found does help us to make these on-our-feet, instantaneous decisions, is the experience we gain from our yoga *practice*, and it all starts with *asana*.

When we overdo the "hard" aspect in our *asana* practice, straining through ambition or competitiveness to get further (which you may have already noticed yourself doing), it drains our energy. We are using more energy than is necessary to accomplish the maximum potential of that posture at that moment. Let's say we are tight in our hamstrings. As we attempt to do the first posture of this chapter, the Lying Down Hamstring Stretch, we will notice that tightness. We want to look "good." So we strain to pull our leg higher. The directions say not to bend the knee, but we don't really notice that. We are uncomfortable with the tightness, so we bend the knee, cheating a little bit, to try and be somewhere we are not and to fog the very clear vision in that moment of what is really true. We don't want truth. We want achievement.

As we learn to pay attention, we can actually *feel* this subtle but very powerful drain on our system. We discover that as we "let go" or back off a bit, and focus a bit more closely, we can actually access more strength! The energy we were wasting through struggling for *more* suddenly becomes available. We relax a bit. I don't mean we go to sleep. I mean we become more present, more tuned into true balance. There is no secret to this. Just follow the instructions — pay attention to the breath, the *drishti*, and the *bandhas* (see next section). The physical effort of getting your attention into present time will slowly bring you to equipoise. And when we become present, for the moment, we are no longer driven by the ego's insatiable desire for more, and we become content with what is. The resistance drops away and we are in touch with true reality — not some imagined state in the future, or some remembered condition of the past. We are really here. We have gained strength through letting go.

RAISING THE BAR WITH THE BANDHAS

Hopefully, you have spent quite a bit of time in your practice by now raising the heat in your body and getting your sweating mechanism turned on. Up to this point, the most fundamental way that we have created this heat (and learned focus) has been through the effort of conscious, static muscular exertion while actually doing the postures. We contracted a muscle and this effort took attention, burned fuel, and heated us up! Then we added the slightly more subtle method of the *ujjayi* breathing, which was, in reality, actually more powerful than just squeezing muscles. I'm quite sure by now you have noticed a strong relationship between the breath and your heat. When you allow the breath to fall off, or forget about it, the heat falls too, and the sweating stops. You might feel like you are cooling down. Since we will now be working with the Seated Postures, on the floor, it's a bit easier to relax a little too much and lose heat. So it is really important to keep the breath going and the appropriate muscle contractions active.

Now we are going to add another mindfulness technique, even more subtle than the breathing, and just as powerful — if not more so. This technique is called a *bandha* or "lock." There are two *bandhas* that we will make use of in our *asana* practice — the first is called *mula* (root) *bandha* and the second is *uddiyana* (to fly upward) *bandha*. The first of these, "root lock," refers simply to a conscious, static contraction of the perineum, a small group of muscles that lies at the floor, or "root" of the pelvis. This lock is engaged by simply squeezing and "lifting" (or consciously contracting) the perineum (to be anatomically correct, we should note that the perineum technically includes the perineal muscle, the anal sphincters and, in women, the vaginal sphincters). The second, "to fly upward lock," refers to a slight physical contraction of the abdominal muscles just a few inches below the navel. To engage this lock, basically, you just pull in your lower belly slightly and lift.

As beginners or even intermediate practitioners, these locks seem to be strictly physical activities, simple muscular contractions that serve to create heat and focus attention and we work hard to "hold" them. This is all correct, but as our practice matures, we recognize that the *bandhas* are — more accurately and more importantly — actually *energetic* contractions, intended to move and uplift *prana*, or energy.

Explaining the *bandhas* is kind of tricky. They aren't things. So we can't really say that *mula bandha* is "located" at the base of the spine. A *bandha* is actually something you *do* to something located in roughly that vicinity!! Although you do begin your work with the "locks" by engaging and holding particular muscles in contraction (like the perineum for *mula bandha*) — and this action does affect the physical body — in principle, a *bandha* actually occurs within what is called a *chakra*, or an "energy center." There are seven *chakras*, which are located within our *energetic* body, and they are spread out along the midline of this energetic body from the base of the spine to the top of the head.

Mula bandha is a conscious activity that is intended to close off or "lock" the 1st or *muladhara chakra* (see box on opposite page for the definition and location of each of the *chakras*). It's kind of like locking your front door at night, so nothing gets in or out. It's the same with *mula bandha*. It keeps energy from escaping. We learn to get in touch with *mula bandha* by first learning to "tighten" the perineum, but eventually we use it to move

SPINNING WHEELS OF LIGHT

According to yoga theory, our physical body is accompanied and surrounded by an electromagnetic field called the energetic body, and within this energetic body, there are seven energy centers, called *chakras*. These energy centers, or *chakras*, are envisioned as spinning wheels of light, and in all actuality, that is exactly what they probably look like if only our perceptual boundaries allowed us to see them. According to yoga philosophy, these seven *chakras*, which increase in their vibrational frequency (spin rate) as you move up from the 1st *chakra* at the base of the spine to the 7th *chakra* at the top of the head.

The seven chakras are:

- 1st *chakra*, called *muladhara* — "the root, or source of our support" — is located at the base of the spine. The color generally associated with this *chakra* is red and its element is Earth.

- 2nd *chakra*, called *svadhishthana* — "place of our origin" — is located a couple of inches below the navel. The color generally associated with this *chakra* is orange and its element is water.

- 3rd *chakra*, called *manipura* — "place where the jewels are kept" — is located at the solar plexus. The color generally associated with this *chakra* is yellow and its element is fire.

- 4th *chakra*, called *anahata* — "that which is ever new; continuously renewing itself" — is located at the heart center. The color generally associated with this *chakra* is green and its element is air.

- 5th *chakra*, called *vishuda* — "purest of the pure" — is located at the notch of the throat. The color generally associated with this *chakra* is blue and its element is space.

- 6th *chakra*, called *ajna* — "command center; the center of the wheel" — is located at the third eye, or point between the eyebrows. The color generally associated with this *chakra* is indigo and its element is light.

- 7th *chakra*, called *sahasrara* — "thousand-petaled lotus" — is located at the crown of the head. The color generally associated with this *chakra* is violet and its element is Consciousness.

and conserve energy. Together, *mula bandha* and the second lock, *uddiyana bandha*, control a form of *prana*, or energy, called *apana*. *Apana* circulates in the lower abdominal area and regulates all movement associated with reproduction and elimination. The nature of *apana* is to move down and out, and you will notice, if you think about it, that all of this lower abdominal "activity" — menstruation, birth, production of eggs and sperm, defecation, urination, and the rest of it, tends to move downward in the body. *Mula bandha* reverses that energy and pulls it up. So, for example, you wouldn't want to be doing *mula bandha* when you were trying to deliver a baby! But as long as you aren't trying to go to the bathroom or give birth, *mula bandha* can be engaged to bring *apana* up! Well why, pray tell, in the world would you want to do that?

The function of both locks is threefold. First, the locks themselves, as we try to initiate their action in the physical body, are actual muscular contractions; they take effort and energy to maintain, and consequently generate heat and contribute to sweating and detoxification. Second, because they take awareness to do and to maintain, both locks serve, along with *drishti* and *ujjayi* breathing as another mindfulness tool. *Mula bandha*, for example, doesn't just happen automatically, the way our leg and back muscles respond mechanically when we want to get up from the couch and walk to the kitchen. In order to hold *mula bandha*, we have to continuously pay attention to it, so in that sense it is a very powerful means for developing mindfulness.

Like *ujjayi* breathing and *drishti*, *mula bandha* is training our mind to be present. Third, because *mula bandha* and *uddiyana bandha* are actually located in the energy body, they are designed to move energy upwards through the *chakras*, raising awareness, and, according to yogic thought, bringing greater lightness and wisdom.

Mula bandha isn't an easy technique to get in touch with and can take a long time to master, as you will see. It's buried down there in the deep recesses of the pelvis — not quite as tangible as the belly muscles, for example. *Uddiyana* is a little easier to "get hold of" but still requires constant vigilance. Once learned, though, both *bandhas* are extraordinarily powerful techniques. *Uddiyana*, especially, drives the breath up into the thoracic cavity by causing the diaphragm to descend, on inhalation, into a reduced space created by the physical pulling in of the abdominal area. This isometric training for the diaphragm and the intercostals (muscles between the ribs) can help to dramatically strengthen these primary respiratory muscles, and as a result, learning to use the *bandhas* is excellent training for anyone with asthma, allergies, or any respiratory limitation.

Mula bandha is also excellent for prostate conditions. For many years I taught private yoga classes in New York City to Michael Korda who, at the time, was editor-in-chief of Simon & Schuster. I had the opportunity to meet Michael shortly after my book *Power Yoga* was published by Simon & Schuster. He saw my book come through his office, was intrigued by the title, and from then on became a regular weekly client. Michael was a dedicated yoga practitioner, and made great progress in the *asanas*. But as a result of an athletic background and years in the Royal Air Force in England, he was tight, so it was not easy for him! In 1996, Michael wrote a book, *Man to Man*, about his experience with prostate cancer, and detailed some of the difficulties men can face following surgery. In our work together, we focused for months and months on the use of *mula bandha* as a tool not only for mindfulness, but as a technique to help him regain continence and full control of the associated prostate equipment. In every posture, I would remind him to engage *mula bandha* and breathe. We worked to strengthen the perineum, as well as to energetically restore the active function and balance of the 2nd *chakra*, which — again, according to yogic thought — actually controls the health of the reproduction organs and leads to healthy reproductive function. Michael regained continence as well as full sexual and urinary function

Since that time, I've worked with other men with similar problems. I think *mula bandha* works so well because it is, on the most fundamental level, strengthening exercise for the perineum. For men, it's similar to the sensation of being on a long road trip, having to pee, but not being able to stop to go to the bathroom, so holding back. The perineal muscle helps to control the flow of urine and semen, so it is an important muscle to develop in connection with restoring full function

to the bladder and the prostate gland, organs often weakened by prostate cancer and surgery. The physical muscular contraction component of the *bandha* gets stronger through use and causes increased blood flow to the area, which promotes healing and return to normal function. I'm not sure if there have been any controlled studies on the use of *mula bandha* for restoration of continence following prostate surgery, but it would certainly be a good research project to set up.

For women, *mula bandha* is similar to the Kegel exercises, the name given to the vaginal contraction exercises often prescribed to pregnant women to strengthen the cervix and vaginal muscles prior to childbirth. As usual, do the best you can with the *mula bandha* techniques. Don't strain. They are not herculean in nature, simply mindful. They can be done easily with a bit of attention. But the point is to patiently, day by day, physically train ourselves as much as possible, to hold these contractions. The energetic component will come slowly. In a strictly classical sense, without the locks, the *practice* isn't "yoga." The mindfulness element is what makes the physical "exercise" yoga. In other words, if you don't pay attention to yourself in your practice, then you can't call your practice yoga.

THE SEATED POSTURES

Okay, let's move on to the Seated Postures. Continue to work with the *ujjayi* breathing and the *drishti*, now seeing if you can begin to incorporate the use of the *bandhas*. Once you develop a sense of them, they are to be added in to the entire practice. In other words, you will be working to be mindful of the *bandhas*, as well as the *drishti* and *ujjayi* breathing in the Sun Salutations and the Standing Postures. You should find, after a bit, that they help with balance, add heat, and give you greater focus and *sthira*, or steadiness! They are theoretically to be held — nonstop — from start to finish of your *asana* routine. However, it will take you many years of practice to accomplish this.

As with the Standing Postures, add on these poses one at a time as you develop strength, endurance, and concentration. Remember, it is imperative that you always leave time at the end of your practice for Relaxation Posture and rest. At whatever point in the sequence you end, lie down and do Knees to Chest Posture (this chapter, page 107). Then stretch your arms directly out to the sides, keeping your shoulders on the floor as best you can. Roll your knees to one side, taking them towards your elbows, and hold there for a few breaths, then change sides. Come back to the center for one more knee to chest hug, and then come into Relaxation Posture (see chapter 3, page 45) and take rest for at least ten minutes.

STICK POSTURE

1. *Inhale*, place the palms on the floor alongside the torso. Flex the thighs and feet, keeping the heels touching the floor. If you are prone to hyperextension at the back of your knees, be especially vigilant about not letting the heels come up off the floor.

2. *Exhale*, lift the spine. Expand the heart. Tuck the head slightly forward. *Drishti* is straight out in front of you. Take 5 breaths. Be mindful of the two *bandhas*. This is a good place to practice them. See if you can hold them for the full 5 breaths, remaining relaxed and focused. Go directly into the next posture.

NOTE: This posture may seem pretty easy, but it is extremely important to learn and to do correctly with strength and awareness. **Stick Posture is the posture that you will return to in between all the Seated Postures, to gather yourself and refocus.**

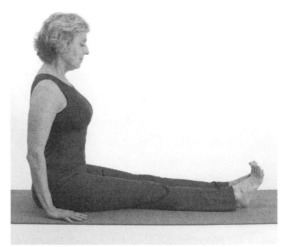

STICK POSTURE

LYING DOWN HAMSTRING STRETCH POSTURE

1. *Inhale*, lie down, with both legs straight out along the floor. Lift the right leg as high as you can and

2. *Exhale*, take hold of the back of the leg, at the calf or behind the knee or thigh.

3. *Inhale* again, and straighten both legs and hold the thigh muscles contracted (you've had practice with this in the Standing Postures). Keeping the head and shoulders on the floor,

4. *Exhale*, bend your elbows, engaging the bicep muscles, and pull the right leg towards your chest. (If this is difficult due to tightness in the back of the legs, then bend your right knee slightly.) Hard press out with both heels, as that helps engage the quadriceps. *Drishti* is at your right knee. Hold for 5 breaths. Again, remember to engage your locks whenever you think of it. After your 5th exhalation,

5. *Inhale*, and then exhale, release the posture, taking your leg back to the floor.

6. *Inhale*, lift the left leg. Repeat instructions for the left side. After your 5th exhalation, *inhale*, and *exhale*, release the posture. Return to Stick Posture. Go directly to the next posture.

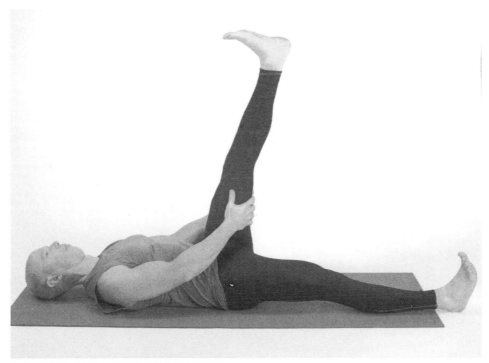

LYING DOWN HAMSTRING STRETCH POSTURE

The Lying Down Hamstring Stretch Posture is a modification of a forward-bending pose, called Intense West Stretch Posture, which is done seated with both legs straight out in front. In this posture, the hands take hold of the toes and then the body bends forward over the extended legs. What happens when people with tight hamstrings or a tight lower back do this posture is that, because of the tightness in the back of the legs or lumbar spine, the pelvis is tipped under, and in order to bend forward, it is necessary for them to round the back excessively and strain to "look" flexible (simulated in photo below). This is wicked awful for the back — especially when it is repeated over a long period of time. However, by doing this lying down, one leg at a time, the back can't round, and that isolates the stretch in the hamstring muscles and protects the back. It is very important to pay attention to the static contraction you are trying to maintain in the quadriceps. The muscles work in pairs, and when the quads are contracted it signals the hamstrings that it is okay to let go and stretch.

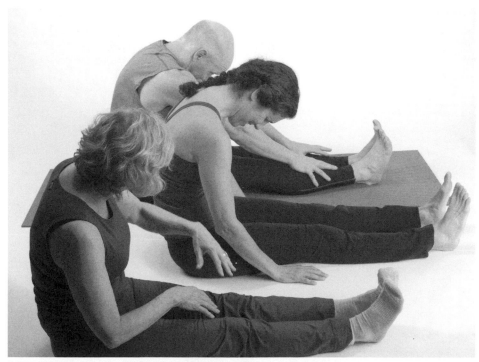

INTENSE WEST STRETCH POSTURE, INCORRECT FORM

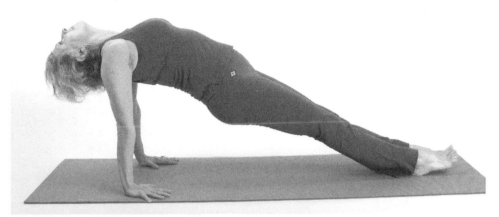

INTENSE EAST STRETCH POSTURE

INTENSE EAST STRETCH POSTURE

From Stick Posture

1. *Inhale* and take your hands behind you, placing them flat on the floor with the fingers pointing towards your body.

2. *Exhale*, raise the torso, and press the hips towards the ceiling. Just lift up as far as you can. If you can and it feels okay for your neck, drop your head all the way back. The *drishti* is at a point behind you. If that bothers your neck, then keep the head up and the chin tucked. In that case, the *drishti* is at your toes. Hold for 5 breaths. After your 5th exhalation, then

3. *Inhale*, and on the exhalation, release the posture, returning to Stick Posture. Go directly to the next posture.

NOTE: If the front of your shoulders are tight, you will probably be able to lift up only a few inches off the floor. That's fine. Do the best you can. Try taking your hands an inch or so farther back, then try again, and see if it is easier. As you stretch out in the shoulders and gain more strength, you will be able to lift higher. Internally rotate the thigh bones, keeping the legs pressed together. Don't hard-point your toes as that can cause the plantar fascia tendon (the bottom of the foot) to cramp. Instead, press out through the balls of your feet. Keep the head up and the chin tucked. (If you can and it is comfortable for you, drop your head back and gaze behind you.)

This posture is totally great for anyone with excessive thoracic (middle back) curvature, osteoporosis in the upper back, and/or tight pectoralis (front of shoulders) muscles. Dropping your head back is not necessarily bad for your neck. It is only bad if it causes you pain or if you have neck issues or high blood pressure, in which case it is recommended that you keep your head forward, gazing at your toes.

VINYASA TO SEATED HALF LOTUS POSTURE

At any point in the practice, you may wish to pop in some connecting movement (*vinyasa*) between the postures, as we did, for example, in the last chapter before and after Fierce Posture, and after the Warrior Postures. This means that instead of just going directly into the next posture, you insert that little *vinyasa* clip from the Sun Salutation.

When you are doing the Seated Postures, this *vinyasa* now involves bending your knees, crossing your ankles, placing your hands on the floor alongside your torso, lifting up your legs (top photo) and torso if you can, then rolling over your feet (middle photo) or if you lift up high enough, swinging your legs underneath you (bottom photo) and stepping them back into the plank position (opposite page, top photo). You then go from push-up position (opposite page, second photo) (*exhale*) to Face Up Dog Posture (*inhale*), and then to Face Down Dog Posture (*exhale*), and then walk or hop your feet back (on an *inhale*) to your hands and sit down again, returning to Stick Posture. Whew! The whole purpose of this little interval is to keep the heat up, develop strength, and reset the body into neutral biomechanical alignment.

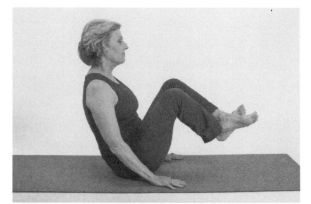

VINYASA 1

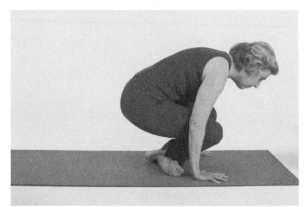

VINYASA 2

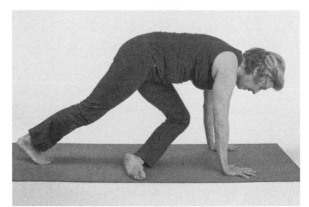

VINYASA 3

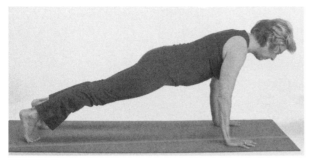

VINYASA 4

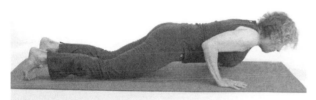

SUN SALUTATION POSITION 4

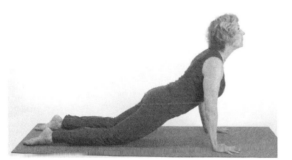

FACE UP DOG POSTURE

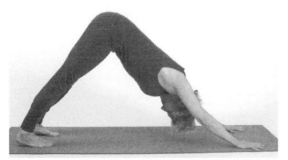

FACE DOWN DOG POSTURE

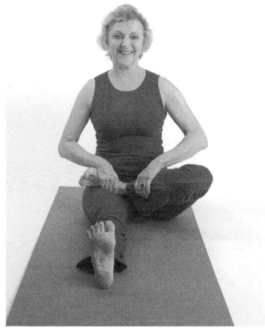

SEATED HALF LOTUS POSTURE

SEATED HALF LOTUS POSTURE

1. *Inhale*, take hold of the right ankle with both hands and placing the foot on the opposite thigh,

2. *Exhale*, pull the heel up and in towards the lower left abdominal quadrant. Engage your arms. Sit up tall, find your *drishti* (straight out in front of you), and take 5 breaths. Once you find your posture, see if you can find stillness and hold *mula* and *uddiyana bandha* for as long as you can keep your attention focused on them, by lifting through the floor of the

pelvis and pulling in the belly. As a general note, you should feel the movement of the breath in the rib cage, not in the belly; the belly shouldn't move. Keeping this awareness will help you to maintain *uddiyana bandha*. If, due to tightness in your hips, you can't bring the heel of your right foot all the way up to the abdomen, then just do the best you can, centering the right ankle on the left thigh and slowly moving it up the thigh bone towards the belly (photo opposite).

3. *Inhale* and *exhale* and release the posture. Repeat the instructions for the left side. Go directly to the next posture, or put in a *vinyasa* as you just did for the posture above. Return to Stick Posture, and then go to the next posture

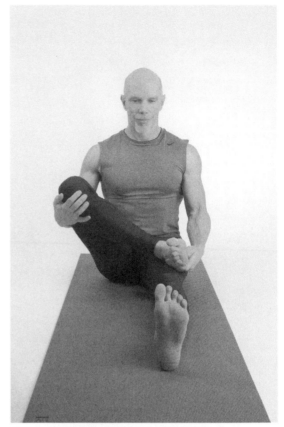

SEATED HALF LOTUS POSTURE, MODIFIED

The principles here are the same as in the standing version of this posture. If getting the foot up into "lotus" position is difficult, just work slowly and patiently, moving closer day by day. Keep your knee up, especially if it bothers you at all, and see if you can swing your knee around to point forward instead of allowing it to point out to the side. If your hips will allow this movement, the heel will be pressing into the belly. If not, do the best you can, pulling the foot in slightly using the strength of your arm. Don't force the knee in any way. Do not even think of bending forward. This movement is designed to stretch the gluteus minimus and gluteus medius muscles — the muscles in the buttocks that abduct the hips and get tight with almost any sport we do. It is often this tightness in these two gluteal muscles that make it easy to injure your knee if you strain. Forget about forcing the knee into half lotus position — open the hips first and the knee will just automatically fall into place! The bandhas *will help you to be mindful and thus, help to prevent injury!*

SEATED TWIST POSTURE

1. *Inhale*, bring your right heel tight up against your right buttock bone, or as close as possible. Make sure your right foot is parallel to the left thigh and flat on the floor, and that you have at least a palm's width of space between your right foot and left thigh. This sounds easy, but most people get sloppy here and have the foot plastered up against the inside of the thigh. Hmmmm, cozy but incorrect.

2. *Exhale*, slide the left leg forward, so that the left hip is slightly more forward than the right hip.

3. *Inhale*, wrap the left arm low around the shin and begin a twist to your right, This shifting of your pelvis, so it is slightly angled to the right (in the direction you are turning) will initiate the twist at the hips, instead of at the lower back. This will take the stress out of the sacroiliac joint as you attempt to rotate the thoracic (middle) spine and turn into the posture.

4. *Exhale*, use the strength in your left arm to pull yourself into the twist. Take the right arm behind you, placing it flat on the floor, which will help to prop you up and keep your spine perpendicular to the floor. *Drishti* is back over your right shoulder. Take 5 breaths.

5. *Inhale*, then *exhale*, release the posture and return to Stick Posture. Repeat the instructions for the left side. Go directly to the next posture.

NOTE: You are working to eventually move your sternum (the chestplate) and left shoulder past your right thigh so that the chest is facing to the right. If you are large-breasted, you might need to lean back first, and try to clear the breasts past the thigh and then move the torso into the leg Most people do not have the rotational flexibility in the thoracic spine to make the full twist. Put your strength into the twist by using your arms to help make the rotation. Don't strain! Be sure to sit up tall, sitting directly on your buttocks bones, and keeping the spine perpendicular to the floor. Try not to lean back, although if you are tight in the hamstrings and/or hips, you will find yourself leaning back a bit.

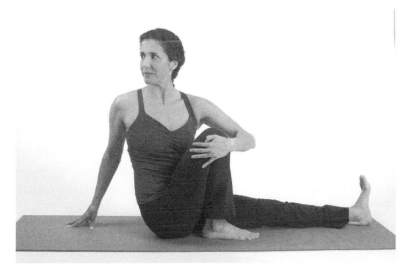

SEATED TWIST POSTURE

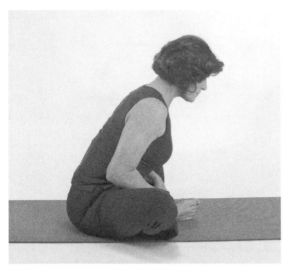

BOUND ANGLE POSTURE, SIDE VIEW

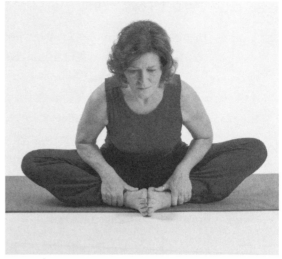

BOUND ANGLE POSTURE

BOUND ANGLE POSTURE

1. *Inhale*, place the soles of the feet together and pull the feet into the groin so that your heels are as close to the perineum as possible. Take hold of your ankles with both hands and extend the spine, sitting up straight, lift the chest, and

2. *Exhale*, bend forward as far as you are able with a straight back (you might not be able to go too far). Do not flex, or round your spine. Don't push on your knees to get them to go to the floor or worry about getting your knees down. They will eventually relax down as the groin muscles let go and the hips open. Keep the elbows tucked in at your sides. You may be really tight in this posture and feel uncomfortable. Be mindful *not* to hunch your shoulders up around your ears or scrunch

down or stick your head out like a turtle. Keep the head in neutral (not forward and not back, not lifting the chin, and not dropping the head) which you can see in the side view of this posture (top photo, left). Go as far as you can. Don't worry. Just breathe (top photo, right). *Drishti* is straight out past the end of your nose. Take 5 breaths. It's really, really important to hold *mula bandha* in this posture, as well as *uddiyana*. The two locks, and especially root lock, will help to prevent you from overstretching.

3. *Inhale*, look up, lift the chest and extend the spine even more, then exhale, release the posture. Take a *vinyasa* or return to Stick Posture. Then, go directly to the next posture.

SEATED ANGLE POSTURE

1. *Inhale*, spread the legs about 90 degrees apart or slightly wider. Grab the shins, ankles, or the back of your knees, or take hold of the big toes with the first two fingers, lift the chest, and look up. Contract the thigh muscles, and here, as in all the *asanas*, really focus on *mula* and *uddiyana bandha*. The hamstrings are very vulnerable in this position to tweaks and tears if you try to strain or overstretch. Holding *mula bandha*, especially, and paying close attention to holding the thighs contracted, prevents injury. It's important!

2. *Exhale*, fold forward as far as possible, which may well be not very far! Hold the spine in extension, as in the last posture. Don't round the back. If you are tight in the hamstrings, this will be a difficult pose. Don't worry about trying to look flexible or getting your head to the floor (if you happen to be flexible enough to do that, then you should know that the head is the very last body part to touch the floor — after the belly and the chest!). *Drishti* is straight out past the end of your nose. Don't drop your head; keep it in alignment with the spine. Hold for 5 breaths (bottom photo, left). Sit up straight and don't round your back (bottom photo, right).

3. *Inhale*, look up and extend even more strongly, squeeze the thighs even more strongly, then *exhale*, and release the posture. Take a *vinyasa* or return to Stick Posture. Then, go directly to the next posture.

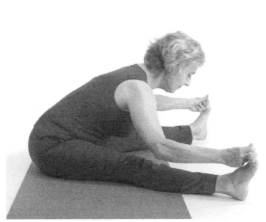

SEATED ANGLE POSTURE

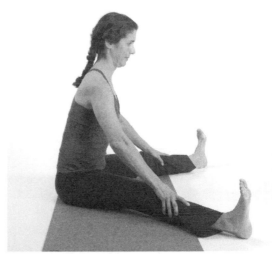

SEATED ANGLE POSTURE

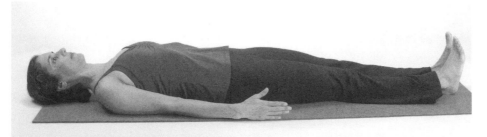

RECLINING MOUNTAIN POSTURE

RECLINING ANGLE POSTURE

1. Lie down, with legs and feet together, feet flexed, and arms at your sides. Prepare for Reclining Angle by coming into a supine version of Mountain Posture. This lying-down "attention" position is called Reclining Mountain Posture (top photo).

2. *Inhale*, raise the legs in the air and separate them as far apart as possible, keep your hips on the floor.

3. *Exhale*, reach up with your arms and take hold of the back of your legs somewhere — behind the calves or knees or ankles. This is the same posture that you just did while sitting, with your legs spread apart, only now you are lying down. *Drishti* is down toward your heart center. Hold for 5 breaths (photo below, left). After your 5th exhalation, bend your knees, cross your ankles, and roll up to a seated position.

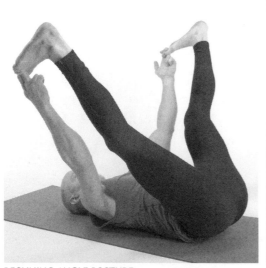

RECLINING ANGLE POSTURE

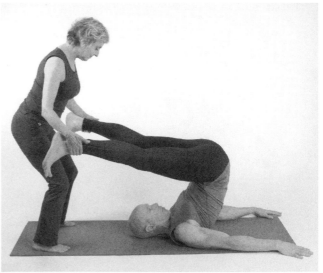

RECLINING ANGLE POSTURE, ADVANCED

If you would like to go a little further into the Reclining Angle Posture, you can take your legs slightly over your head, using a wall or friend to prop your feet on (opposite page, photo bottom right). This additional stretch will increase the angle of flexion at the back of your neck and at the lower back. How far you go depends on how flexible your hamstrings are, because if they are tight it will limit how far you can safely take your legs over your head without overbending/stressing the spine. As you become more pliable, you can increase this angle slowly. Pay attention. Don't just flop into this.

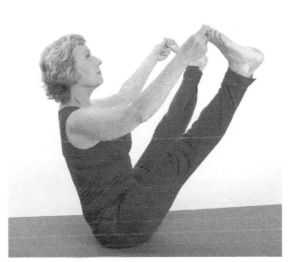

BALANCED ANGLE POSTURE

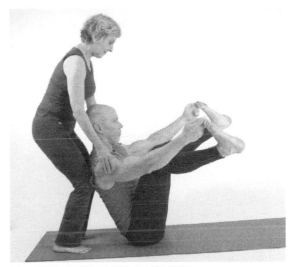

BALANCED ANGLE POSTURE, MODIFIED

BALANCED ANGLE POSTURE

1. *Inhale*, from a seated position, bend your knees, and take hold or your big toes with the first two fingers on each hand.

2. *Exhale*, see if you can lean back a bit, lift your feet off the floor, and extend your legs and then come to balance. If your hamstrings are tight, then keep your knees bent slightly or hold your legs behind your knees or calves, instead of at the toes (top photo, right). If you can extend all the way, then hold in that position. *Drishti* is up. Hold for 5 breaths. After your 5th exhalation, release the posture. Bend your knees, cross your ankles, lift up and take a *vinyasa*. (Jump or step back to push-up position, then Face Up Dog, Face Down Dog, and hop back or step through to sitting.) Lie down in Reclining Mountain Posture (top photo, opposite page). Go directly to the next posture.

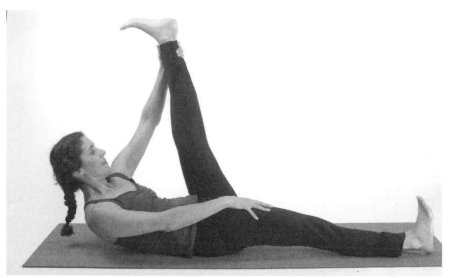

LYING DOWN HAND TO LEG POSTURE A

LYING DOWN HAND TO LEG POSTURE A

1. *Inhale*, raise the right leg and take hold of it with your right hand, wherever you can — back of the knee, or thigh, or ankle. Place your left hand on your left thigh.

2. *Exhale*, lift your head and shoulders up off the floor, taking your nose toward your knee. *Drishti* is at your toes. Hold for 5 breaths. After your 5th exhalation,

3. *Inhale*, lower your head and shoulders to the floor and

4. *Exhale*, open the leg out to the side. This will take you right into the next posture.

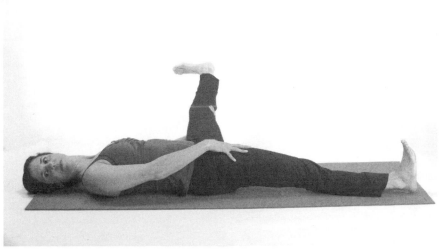

LYING DOWN HAND TO LEG POSTURE B

LYING DOWN HAND TO LEG POSTURE B

1. *Drishti* is to your left (the opposite direction from the leg out to the side.) Be sure to try to keep both legs straight — pressing out hard through the heels of both feet. You might need to re-adjust your hand position as the leg opens out to the side. This is fine — just don't bend your knee. Keep the quads engaged! Hold for 5 breaths,

2. *Inhale*, raise the leg back up to center, and

3. *Exhale*, take your nose up toward your knee.

4. *Inhale*, lower the head again and

5. *Exhale*, release the leg and return to Reclining Mountain Posture.

6. Repeat this entire sequence (Postures A and B) for the left side (shown in photos opposite and above).

BRIDGE POSTURE

From Reclining Mountain Posture, bring your feet up towards your buttocks bones. Separate your feet about hip-width apart and keep your feet parallel and flat on the floor.

1. *Inhale*, lift the buttocks off the floor, pressing up, and lace your fingers together underneath your torso.

2. *Exhale*, straighten the arms and squeeze the shoulder blades together, stretching the front of your shoulders and working the shoulder blades towards one another.

Drishti is at your heart center. Take 5 breaths. After your 5th exhalation,

3. *Inhale*, and then *exhale* and come down out of the posture. Bend your knees, cross your ankles, and roll up to a seated position. Go through the connecting *vinyasa* (jump back into push-up position, do Face Up Dog Posture, Face Down Dog Posture,) and from Face Down Dog, lie face down. This will take you to the next posture.

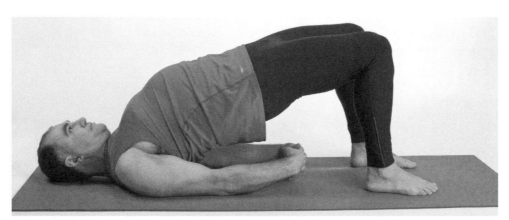

BRIDGE POSTURE

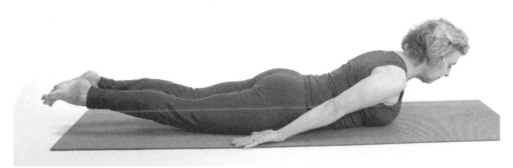

LOCUST POSTURE A

LOCUST POSTURE A

This posture begins the back therapy portion of the *asana* sequence.

1. *Inhale*, arms back along your sides, palms facing up, feet together, chin on the floor.

2. *Exhale*, raise your head, shoulders, and legs into the air. Keep your legs and feet touching each other. Press the back of the hands down into the floor (top photo).

Drishti is straight out in front of you. Keep the head in neutral. Check your *bandhas*! Hold for 5 breaths. After your 5th exhalation, go directly to Locust Posture B unless you need a break between these two, in which case, *inhale*, then *exhale*, and release. Then reposition your hands, as described, for the next posture, and go on.

LOCUST POSTURE B

1. *Inhale*, and if possible, without coming down from Locust Posture A, shift your hand position. Bend the elbows, place the hands flat on the floor, with fingers pointing forward, and then slide your hands back until the wrists are directly under the elbows. Everything else stays the same.

2. *Exhale*, settle in — legs and torso still lifted. Or if you came back down to the floor after Locust Posture A, then lift back up again (photo below). *Drishti* is the same as for Posture A — straight ahead. Find stillness. Remember to hold the perineum lifted and the belly pulled in. It is easy to forget once you begin "back bending," but it becomes even more important to hold the belly in as it helps to lengthen the spine and prevent excess compression in the lower back. Take 5 breaths. After your 5th exhalation, *inhale*, then *exhale* and release the posture. Go directly into

3. *Inhale*, Face Up Dog Posture and

4. *Exhale*, Face Down Dog Posture, and go directly into next posture.

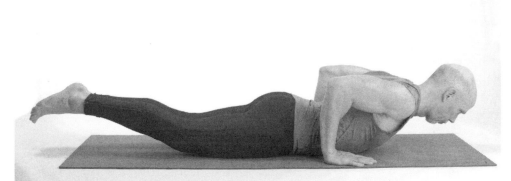

LOCUST POSTURE B

BOW POSTURE — OPTIONAL (MORE ADVANCED)

1. *Inhale* as you bend your knees and reach back and grab your ankles. Dorsiflex your feet (to remind you, that means press out through the heels and flex the toes toward the shins), and keep your legs and feet together, or else keep your legs and feet separated, but parallel!

2. *Exhale*, lift the legs and upper torso. Tip forward slightly, so that the weight is forward toward the stomach (above the waist). Try to straighten your legs, pushing them away from your head. This will help to open the front of the chest, the pectoralis muscles at the front of the shoulders, and the heart center. *Drishti* is straight out in front of you. Take 5 breaths. After your 5th exhalation, *inhale* again, and then *exhale* and release the posture, returning to prone position.

3. *Inhale*, push up into Face Up Dog Posture,

4. *Exhale*, push back into Face Down Dog Posture, and then from there, return to Stick Posture. Go directly to the next posture.

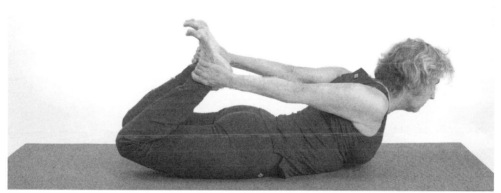

BOW POSTURE, OPTIONAL

In my workshops, I can say keep your feet and legs together a kabillion times and for some reason nobody listens. It is really, really important that you either 1) keep your legs superglued together, or 2) if you need to separate your knees, then you need to separate your feet. Some teachers teach this posture with feet together and knees apart. I disagree with this alignment, as it compresses (instead of creating spaciousness, which most of us need) in the sacroiliac joints.

HERO POSTURE

1. *Inhale*, kneel down, separating your knees about hip-width apart. Spread your feet wide enough to sit between them,

2. *Exhale*, go ahead and sit. If this hurts your knees, don't do it. Keep your feet parallel to one another, with all 10 toes on the floor (photo below, left) — don't allow your feet to flange out to the sides. If you are tight in the tops of your feet or your hips, you might not be able to sit all the way down between your feet or point your feet straight back. If that is the case, place a pillow or block or bolster under your butt, which will enable you to correctly align the feet, ease pressure on your knees, and make you more comfortable (photo below, right). Take

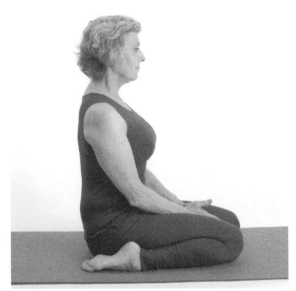

HERO POSTURE

5 breaths in this posture. *Drishti* is straight ahead in front of you. Go directly to the next posture.

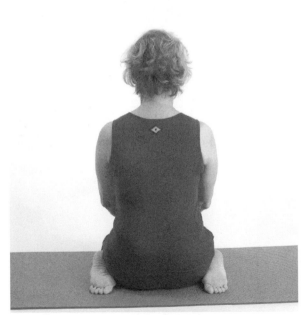

HERO POSTURE

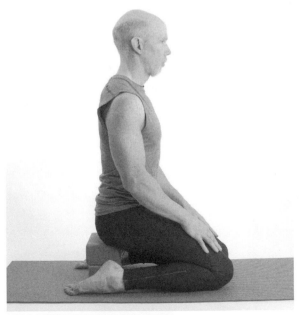

HERO POSTURE WITH BLOCK ASSIST

CAMEL POSTURE

From the kneeling position,

1. *Inhale*, take your hands back on the floor behind you. Place them flat on the floor with the fingers pointing towards you.

2. *Exhale*, lift the hips in the air — press your hips forward, stretching the quadriceps and if you can, allow the head to hang back. If this is not comfortable for your neck, keep the head forward. *Drishti* is straight back, if your head is back; if your head is up, *drishti* is straight out in front of you. Hold for 5 breaths. (photo below, left). If this is a little scary for you, have a buddy support you behind your shoulder blades (not behind the lower back) as you see in the photo below, right. After your 5th exhalation,

3. *Inhale*, and *exhale* and release the posture. At this point, it's probably a good idea to go through a *vinyasa* to stretch out the legs and take any kinks out of your knees. From Face Down Dog Posture, go directly to next posture.

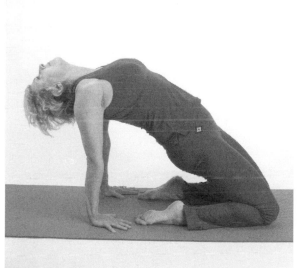

CAMEL POSTURE

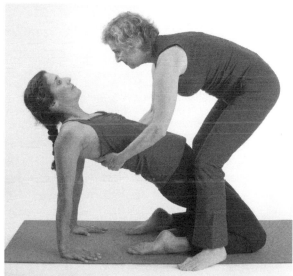

CAMEL POSTURE, WITH ASSIST

HORSE POSTURE

This posture and the next one are excellent stretches for opening the shoulders and pretty good for helping to rehabilitate almost any shoulder injury. So if tight shoulders or an old injury are an issue for you or if you have had shoulder surgery, I would spend a bit of extra time with these. Remember, if your injury or surgery is recent, don't push the stretch. Wait until the healing process gets going, and then little by little, increase the intensity, to prevent scar tissue from forming and tightness from setting into the injury site. This really requires a lot of awareness to get the balance right as to how much to push and how much to back off — so pay attention. Remember, hard and soft!

1. *Inhale*, as you step your right foot forward, placing it between your hands and

2. *Exhale*, and gently lower the left knee to the floor. You may flatten the back foot or keep the toes (pointed under) on the floor.

3. *Inhale*, place the right elbow in the crook of the left elbow and wrap your left hand and arm around the right forearm. See if you can touch the base of your right palm with your left fingers. Keep the forearms perpendicular to the floor and gently raise the arms, taking the hands and arms straight up as much as possible. This is great therapy for the shoulders and the four muscles in the shoulder that comprise

what is referred to as the "rotator cuff," especially the teres minor muscle, which helps to laterally rotate the arm.

4. *Exhale*, lean into this now by lunging slightly forward. *Drishti* is up at the hands. Hold for 5 breaths.

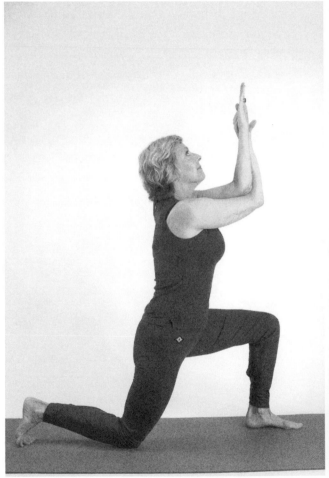

HORSE POSTURE

5. *Inhale*, then exhale and release the posture. Go through a *vinyasa* (push-up posture, Face Up Dog Posture, Face Down Dog Posture) and repeat the instructions for the left side, or you can choose to leave out the *vinyasa* here and simply reverse your feet and change sides. Then work the left side. After completing the left side, though, it's important to run through the *vinyasa* sequence below in order to set your hips and shoulders back to neutral.

6. *Inhale*, then exhale and release the posture.

7. *Inhale*, take the hands to the floor.

8. *Exhale*, step back into your push-up.

9. *Inhale*, Face Up Dog Posture.

10. *Exhale*, Face Down Dog Posture. Step your feet up to your hands and sit down. Come into Stick Posture. Go directly to the next posture.

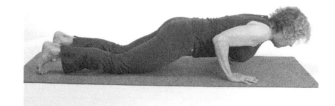

PUSH-UP POSTURE

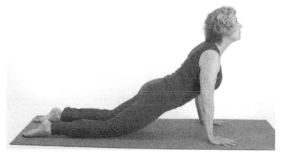

FACE UP DOG POSTURE

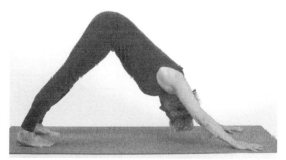

FACE DOWN DOG POSTURE

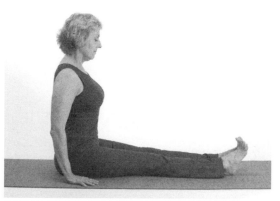

STICK POSTURE

COW'S FACE POSTURE A

From Stick Posture, bend your knees and cross the right knee over the left knee, folding your feet back alongside your hips. Be careful not to sit on your left foot with the right side of your buttocks. Make sure the left foot is clear of your butt . If you are tight in the hips, it will very quickly become apparent that this is rather difficult. This is an excellent posture to do for tight or misaligned hips. It won't feel great at first if you are tight, or bound up in the hips (2nd *chakra*). Do the best you can. Gaze down at the floor. Take 5 breaths. After your last exhalation,

1. *Inhale*, fold your hands over your right knee.

2. *Exhale*, send the energy down through the right buttock bone, anchoring it to the floor. Try not to let it lift up. *Drishti* is down at the floor. Take 5 breaths. After your last exhalation, release your hands.

3. *Inhale*, as you lift your right arm in the air, bend your elbow, and drop your right hand behind your back, along your spine. This will take you to the next posture, which is the same as what we just did, but with a different arm position.

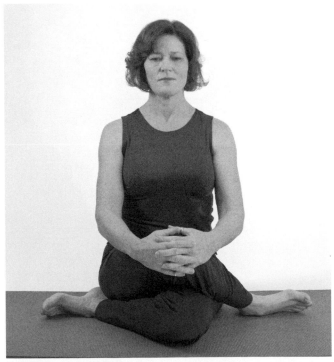

COW'S FACE POSTURE A

COW'S FACE POSTURE B

1. *Inhale*, then *exhale*, take your left hand and push your right elbow back slightly, stretching out the right tricep muscles. *Drishti* stays the same. Hold this for a couple of breaths. Then

2. *Inhale*, then exhale, and let go of your right elbow, take the left arm down and move it behind your back and go to the next posture.

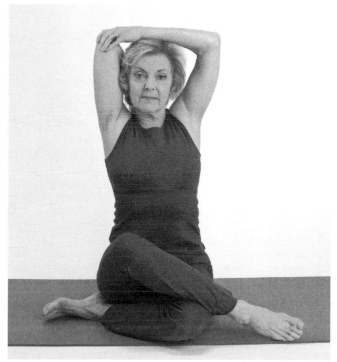

COW'S FACE POSTURE B

COW'S FACE POSTURE C

1. *Inhale*, then *exhale*, reach up and try to clasp the fingers of your right hand with the fingers of your left hand behind your back. If you can't reach use a towel or sock or strap to connect your hands, slowly working them closer together (photo below). Pull the right elbow back as best you can. *Drishti* is up. Hold for 5 breaths. Release your arms, place your hands on the floor in front of you, then bend forward (ugh!) and hold here for 5 breaths (bottom photo right, opposite page).

2. *Inhale*, then exhale and release the posture. Change sides and repeat the instructions for Cow's Face Posture A, B, and C on the other side. From here you may choose to simply lie down in Reclining Mountain Posture or take a *vinyasa*. From Face Down Dog Posture, step through to sitting, coming into Stick Posture. Go directly to the next posture.

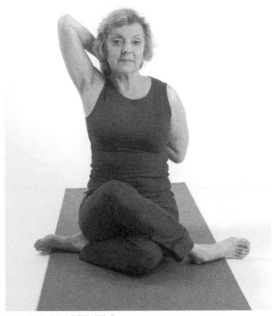

COW'S FACE POSTURE C

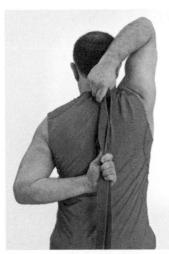

COW'S FACE POSTURE C WITH STRAP ASSIST

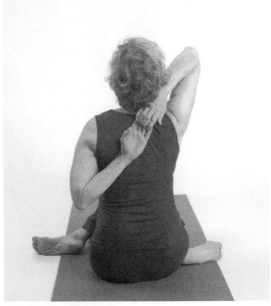

COW'S FACE POSTURE C

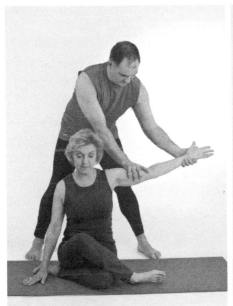

COW'S FACE POSTURE C

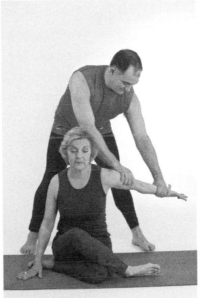

COW'S FACE POSTURE C

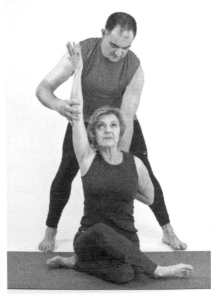

COW'S FACE POSTURE C

The photos at top and bottom left illustrate the way in which a certified professional yoga teacher can mindfully assist you in mastering Cow's Face Posture C.

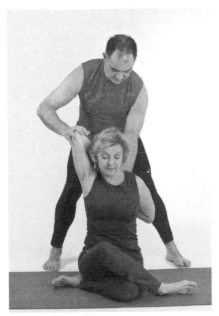

COW'S FACE POSTURE C

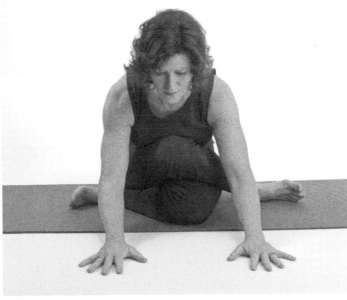

COW'S FACE POSTURE C

BRIDGE POSTURE

We did this posture a short while ago, but will repeat it here now.

1. *Inhale*, lie down, bend your knees and bring your feet up towards your buttocks bones. Separate your feet about hip-width apart and keep your feet parallel and flat on the floor.

2. *Exhale*, lift the buttocks off the floor, pressing up, and lacing your fingers together underneath your torso.

3. *Inhale*, then exhale, straighten the arms and squeeze the shoulder blades together, stretching the front of your shoulders and working the shoulder blades towards one another. *Drishti* is at your heart center. Take 5 breaths. After your 5th exhalation,

4. *Inhale*, then exhale and come down out of the posture. Come into Reclining Mountain Posture.

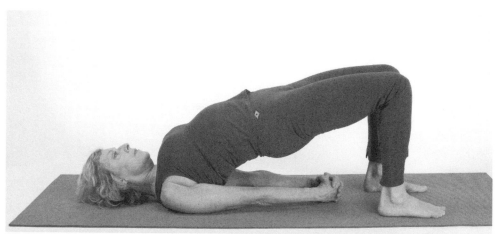

BRIDGE POSTURE

KNEES TO CHEST POSTURE

This is an excellent, therapeutic position for almost all lower back pain. Here we are using it as a counter-pose to the three back-bending, back-therapy postures.

1. *Inhale*, bring your knees to your chest.

2. *Exhale*, take hold of your knees with your hands and pull your knees into your chest, lift the head and shoulders, if you can, tucking your nose into the knees. If this strains your neck, then keep your head, shoulders, and back on the floor.

3. *Drishti* is straight out in front of you. Take 5 breaths. After your last exhalation, release the posture and if you are ending your practice here, then go directly to Relaxation Posture. Otherwise, take a *vinyasa* and return to Stick Posture, then go to the next posture.

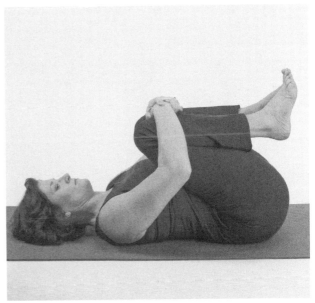

KNEES TO CHEST POSTURE

RECLINING MOUNTAIN POSTURE

1. From Stick Posture, lie down. Bring your feet together and flex them, place your arms at your sides. Keep the eyes open. This is just like Mountain Posture, only you are lying down. *Drishti* is straight out in front of you. Take 5 breaths in this position. After your last exhalation you will go directly to the first posture in chapter 6.

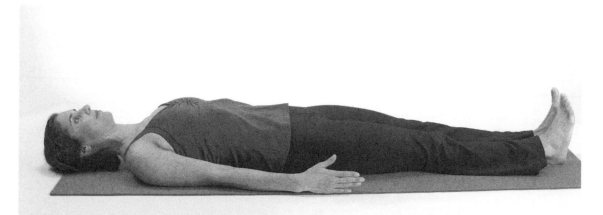

RECLINING MOUNTAIN POSTURE

This completes the chapter on the Seated Postures. Work through them slowly. As with the Standing Postures, add them on to your practice little by little, one at a time. Even though the copy says "go directly to the next posture," that is referring to what you will eventually do in this 40-minute practice, once you have learned correct alignment for the postures and are able to move through the sequence, one after another, without interruption or distraction.

If you have just finished working your way through this chapter, then you will end your practice now with rest. After the last posture, you can continue to the next chapter or you can close out and prepare for Relaxation Posture by doing Lying Down Spinal Twist Posture. Take your knees, side to side, hold for a few breaths on each side, and then come into Relaxation Posture (see page 45). Rest here for at least 10 minutes.

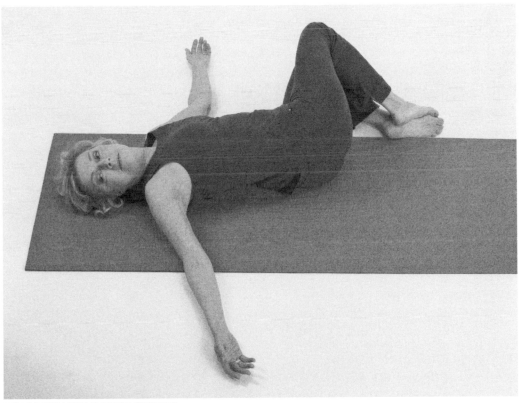

LYING DOWN SPINAL TWIST POSTURE

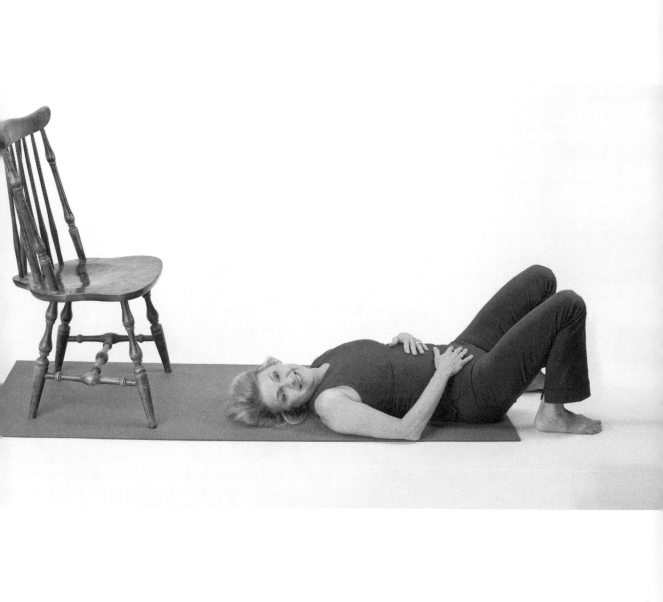

Chapter 6 COOLING DOWN

Coming to Balance

All aspects of our yoga practice should serve us *therapeutically*. A particular posture can act as *therapy* for the back or an injured shoulder, for example. But you may be wondering, "What exactly does that mean? How is this going to be therapeutic for me?"

I think there are unlimited ways in which our yoga practice can be therapeutic and curative and these can be different for everyone — depending on why a person started yoga in the first place and what it is they are looking to fix. Whether it is to reduce the severity of the symptoms of menopause or regain continence after prostate surgery, it is more than likely — as I have frequently mentioned — that a yoga practice, whether *asana*, breath work, or meditation, can be helpful. Some benefits are strictly physical, such as the restructuring of biomechanical or energetic alignment or the restorative effects of *tapas*. Some are more mental, like relieving stress through the conscious breathing technique or training the mind to focus on the present, and thus limiting anxiety and the debilitating effects of stress related disease. Still others are less tangible, where the effects simply make themselves apparent through general feelings of transformation — resulting in a deeper spiritual connection to Self, or greater peace of mind.

But whether we stretch out our hamstrings or slow down our mind, find flexibility or find contentment, I think it is important that we know that all our work in *yoga*, whether *asana*, conscious breathing, meditation, community service, or any mindful activity, really should be beneficial for us. If it isn't helping us, it isn't yoga.

The less tangible, or more spiritual ways in which we change (and it generally seems to be for the better) are a little more difficult to list because they are, well, intangible. If we try to describe our sense of connection to what we might call God, or Great Spirit, or The One, it may be a little hard to talk about without sounding like a proselytizing fanatic! We can talk about our sense of connection to community, though, and how yoga can take us from being self-absorbed to being a little more conscious, a little more aware of what is going on around us, and a little more caring about others.

Now that you have worked your way through the major portion of the *asana* practice, let's take a closer look as to how this system might begin to work as therapy for you. What *are* the important elements that make what we are doing here "therapeutic"? First of all, the practice of *asana* moves us towards balance between strength and flexibility. You have probably already discovered, as you have been practicing, that if you were too tight or too flexible, without being equally flexible and strong, you were most likely out of balance and at risk of injury, if you were not already injured. To be *therapeutic* our practice must be balanced between the stretching and contracting of our muscles. Remember, this isn't a book just about "stretching!"

Our practice also needs to harmonize forward and backward bending. Almost everything we do in life is about bending forward slightly or a lot — driving, eating, lovemaking (for the most part — there are exceptions!), shopping, sitting at a desk, cooking, reading, sleeping, playing with children, vacuuming, gardening, and so forth. It's also comforting and primal to bend forward and curl up. As scary and uncomfortable as it might be, it is important to bend backwards once in awhile. That is why the postures that come later in this chapter that I refer to as the "back therapy" postures are so important to this sequence. They have a balancing and beneficial effect on the body, and help to strengthen the spine and counteract the degenerative tendency of the thoracic curve in our upper back to increase as we grow older. It also stretches out the front of the body — in yoga we say it *opens* the heart center — resulting in changes you can only experience and can't really talk about!

We also need to balance standing upright with being upside down. In this chapter we will explore the early beginning of inverted postures. While we won't exactly do any full inversion, Reclining Angle Posture, (the lying down posture that we did in the last chapter with our legs over our head) begins the inversion process. In this chapter we will modify Shoulder Stand in a similar way, where we raise our legs up over our head, but don't elevate all the way up into full Shoulder Stand Posture. Many people in yoga classes jump into the full inversion postures without adequate preparation when they see others doing them, and end up injured. That is why, in *Boomer Yoga*, I have chosen to include only the modified introductions to these postures, rather than the full postures.

Turning upside down is an invigorating and restorative way to sort of "drain" tension and toxins from the legs, the lower torso, and the major organs, and assist with venous blood return to the heart. According to yogic thought, this helps to dislodge toxins that get "stuck" in the dark corners of the liver, lungs, intestines, etc., and clear out the mental cobwebs. But before you go to a yoga class and get too excited about jumping into a head stand, keep in mind that there are contraindications for the complete inverted postures. If you have untreated high blood pressure, detached retina, any eye condition where increased pressure would be dangerous, neck injuries or misalignments, or any questions about whether or not you should be doing any of the full-on inverted yoga postures (not included in this book!), I would strongly recommend not doing them at all.

FACING PAIN

I think, and so do most of the orthopedists

I have talked to, that the most important thing to do in dealing with osteoarthritis, for example, or when coming back from knee or shoulder surgery or hip replacement, is to *keep moving* in a non-stressful way. But what often happens, is that if we are in pain, as is most likely to occur with arthritis, or if we find our movement limited, as can happen after most any surgery or illness, our tendency is to slow down and move less. And little by little, over time, we become less fit and less active and gradually we start to feel *older*!

What to do? How can we avoid this slow decline? Well to start, we can do just what we have been doing — our *asana* practice. "But it's uncomfortable," you might say.

When I come face to face with this fear of dealing with discomfort, I remind myself that I have a choice. I can deal with it now, on my own terms — in other words, I can move back and forth between the comfortable and the discomfortable — deciding for myself just where to hang out. Or I can deal with it later. But if I don't face it now — whether it is to stretch out, or dislodge toxins, or regain range of motion, or sit still for another twenty minutes, then I will face it later in life, and most likely at that point, I won't have a choice. Look, we all will die some day. But we want to have the healthiest death possible.

STAYING YOUNG

Yoga opens up our joints, creating space in the shut down or compressed areas of old injuries, and making room for circulation of intracel-lular fluids, carrying nutrition in and toxins out. This has a strong anti-inflammatory effect, which is an added health benefit that may very well be the most important of all. Inflammation is one of the greatest contributors to aging, taking a toll on all the systems of the body. The conventional wisdom is that if we can prevent and stop inflammation, we can prevent and stop the signs of aging, or at least slow it down.

I can think of three basic ways to do this and the yoga lifestyle pops up in all of them. The first is through appropriate physical movement — and *asana* serves us as some of the most suitable movement going. Yoga may not be aerobic in the way that running is, but it is *aerobic* in that yoga is practiced "in the presence of oxygen," which is the definition of "aerobic." It does strengthen our heart and lungs, and it doesn't have the detrimental effect of the pounding, that is associated with running, which tends to *create* inflammation.

The second way is through some form of stress management, like breathing and meditation, and again we find the yoga methodology playing an important role, which I will discuss in chapters 7 and 8.

Lastly, a nourishing, anti-inflammatory diet is critical in keeping us young, healthy, and active, and the yogic pattern of eating has long advocated the anti-inflammatory benefits of whole foods — prepared from scratch — such as organic fruits and vegetables, whole grains and legumes, and essential fatty acids.

ADDING TO THE MIX
ELEVEN THINGS TO DO BESIDES *ASANA* THAT WILL KEEP YOU YOUNG

Yoga practice extends from sun-up to sun-down and on into the night. So when we are not doing *asana*, what are we doing that can be called "yoga"? Well hopefully, everything we do can be called our *yoga practice*, but more specifically, what exactly are some things we can do besides our *asana* practice that will be constructive from a therapeutic point of view for our mental and physical and spiritual well-being? Well, it is going to be different for everyone. But there are a number of things that work across the board. And I like to get (at least) most of them in every day

We can **walk**. I walk almost every day. Whether it is cloudy and raining, clear, sunny and gorgeous, or cold and snowing — to be out in it is great. Once you get out, the act of being outside in Nature always lifts your spirits. Remember, our *practice* is to be mindful with what *is* 24/7.

In the summer I also **ride my bike or swim** from time to time. I used to run and loved it. But what I found is that for most people, including me, we aren't perfectly aligned well enough — either because of genetic imbalance or as a result of injury over our lifetime — to sustain running without slowly making our misalignments worse. As a teacher of *asana*, I've worked with thousands upon thousands of runners, and have found that most of them are adding to their misalignment through their running. They may be strengthening their heart and lungs, which is great, but their biomechanical structure is slowly suffering. Yoga can reverse this tendency, but only if it is regularly practiced.

What else? We can **breathe consciously** — whether walking, sitting, washing dishes, or riding on the bus or in our car — *Conscious Breathing*, as we talk about in the next chapter, reduces stress and calms us down. It gets us in touch with the beauty of this moment — whether it is challenging or not!! Try it now — just take a deep *ujjayi* breath. How does that feel? It gets you here — in touch with your body — your mind plugs into the body and you feel whole, complete — for a moment. A good thing.

Staying healthy and living long involves more than just doing *asana* and breathing and walking. It involves cultivating a balanced awareness of what it is we need to do to maintain our health and vitality. So what might that be — well it could include things like **getting enough sleep**, at least eight hours per day. There are tons of articles written in the popular magazines about the deleterious effects of sleep deprivation. Getting enough sleep is essential and part of our *yoga practice*. You don't run on overdrive, trying to do eighteen things at once, working eighteen hours a day, to get "somewhere," if you are *practicing* yoga. You are in balance. You are in touch with what your body needs. When you sleep, you sleep. You already are "somewhere"; you are here.

Not smoking is probably another good item to add to our list. Smoking will definitely cut down on your longevity — whether you do *asana* or not. Some of you reading this may be smokers. It's a choice we make. But you should know, it limits you and if it hasn't already, it will at some point in the future. Doing *asana* seems to slowly eliminate our desire to do or be around anything that limits us in any way. Don't fret. Eventually your desire to smoke will fall away. Just keep *practicing*.

What else is a simple addition to well being? How about to **eat fruit and a colorful salad every day**. I'm very big on "colorful" salads — beets, carrots, different lettuces, red peppers, red cabbage, pomegranate seeds, local tomatoes (in August and September only), and I load up on berries year round — raspberries, blueberries, strawberries, and blackberries when they are in season, and when they aren't, I turn to my frozen supply. I eat bananas even though they come from rather far away (from where I live) and are a little high in sugar, they make smoothies really yummy. I eat apples and pears in the fall, which are local and seasonal; and oranges and grapefruit in the winter, which aren't exactly local or seasonal, so I am grateful for the little bit of extra energy to get them to where I'm at. And I get to eat mangos and papayas on our yoga trips to the Caribbean every year.

Don't eat too much. Overeating is a way of life in the U.S., and it takes its toll on us — it shortens our life in terms of wearing out our processing plant more quickly, creating obesity, and generally overloading and clogging the system. Last night I was at the local movie house and I just could not believe the size of the cups of soda and popcorn that people were lugging around. Wow, it would take two or three yoga stomachs to hold all that stuff. **Mindful eating** involves not just "portion control" but quality

control as well — not too much caffeine, not too much sugar, not too much junk — maybe no caffeine for some of us, maybe no sugar, maybe no junk. No junk is probably always a good idea. Junk is just some marketing guy's idea of how to make money. Give up junk. You'll make yourself and the world a better place. And the people employed in the "junkyards" can become organic farmers.

Call a friend. It feels good to make time for others. Don't just call when you want something, or need to whine about something to someone. Call to make contact. Plan an activity, a vacation. Schedule some time together — a movie, a tea break, a reading date, something community oriented that will benefit your neighborhood.

And finally, **relax**. Funny, people look at my travel schedule and think I'm on this frantic pace and always think they are being helpful by telling me to slow down or take time for myself. But I always take time to relax, to make time to stop and appreciate the moment, either through meditation, or walking with my dogs, or working in the garden, or lying on the couch in the early evening watching *The Daily Show*, or having dinner and **a glass of red wine** with friends.

Life goes so quickly. Every moment is a gift. Sounds corny, but once you really understand how to get in touch with that *moment* you see how profound that idea really is. Life slows down, you become more grateful and appreciative of what you have, and you forget about getting old and aging, because there is no "future," no "aging," there is only "here" — the only place you can ever truly be.

CLOSING OUT

We have now come to the last postures in the boomer yoga sequence. Once you get to this point in your *practice*, you have worked long enough with the preliminary postures and on developing your strength and flexibility to be able to do these Closing Postures easily and safely. So far, you've been adding postures to your practice just a few at a time. Now, however, you need to add all eight of the following Closing Postures all at once. Generally this group of postures will end your practice. However, there may be times when, due to time restraint or other circumstances, you will simply do Sun Salutations, or Sun Salutations and the Standing Postures. Then you might skip to the very last three postures, Forward Bend Easy Posture, Easy Posture, and Lifted Easy Posture (which is not easy!).

THE CLOSING POSTURES

HALF SHOULDER STAND POSTURE

Lie down in Reclining Mountain Posture. This is your preparation for Half Shoulder Stand and serves to get you centered and grounded and energized for the posture. Take five breaths in this position. Before you begin Half Shoulder Stand Posture.

1. *Inhale*, lift legs in the air and then

2. *Exhale*, and lift your hips about half-way up in the air if possible. Support your back with your hands. There should be no strain on your neck.

3. *Inhale*, and *exhale*, straighten your legs. *Drishti* is straight up in the air. Hold here for 10 breaths. After your last exhalation, go directly into the next posture

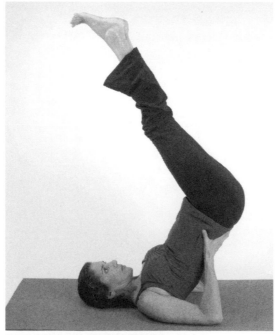

HALF SHOULDER STAND POSTURE

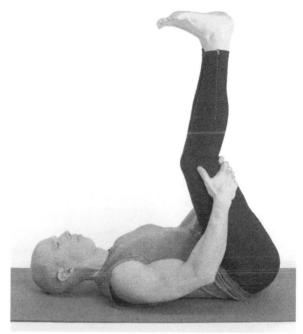

HALF SHOULDER STAND POSTURE, MODIFIED

If Half Shoulder Stand Posture proves to be too much stress on your wrists, or if you have any kind of eye problem that would respond poorly to increased pressure, or if you have high cholesterol or untreated high blood pressure, this lifting of the hips is a bit too much strain. In that case, keep your hips on the floor and just raise your legs. If your hamstrings are tight, this won't be so comfortable and you will struggle a bit to try and hold your legs up there, so in that case, bend your knees and take hold of the back of your legs with your hands. Remember, keep your head, shoulders, and back on the floor. If you are flexible enough to raise your legs 90 degrees or more, without bending your knees, this will be a very relaxing and effortless position and you can place your hands on the floor alongside your body.

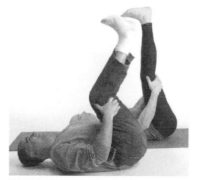

HALF SHOULDER STAND POSTURE, MODIFIED

KNEES TO EARS POSTURE

This is a modification of the traditional Knees to Ears Posture which is done by taking the legs up and over the head to the floor. In that posture, the buttocks are all the way up in the air and the knees bend and reach to the floor alongside the ears. It's a great posture if you are flexible, especially in the hamstrings, have no neck or lower back injuries, and no high blood pressure or heart conditions or any disease of the eye where increased pressure would be injurious. I felt it would be safer and far more appropriate to include a modification of that posture here, and then if you go on with your yoga, you can always learn this posture safely from a skilled teacher.

1. *Inhale*, bend your knees and lower your legs to your chest.

2. *Exhale*, separate your legs and either continue to support your back with your hands (photo below) or take hold of your calves or feet with your hands. Using your abdominals, try to pull your knees down and toward your ears. Keep your head on the floor. This stretches out the lower and middle back. *Drishti* is straight in front of you or at your heart center. Take 5 breaths in this position.

3. *Inhale* and *exhale*, roll down and out of this posture and come into Reclining Mountain Posture. Go directly into the next posture.

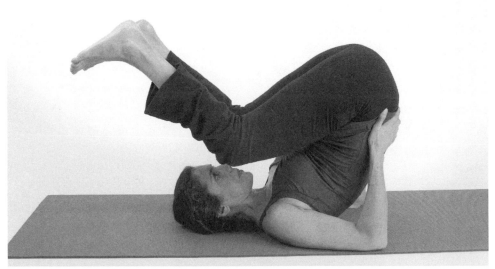

KNEES TO EARS POSTURE

FISH POSTURE

1. *Inhale*, bend your knees and cross your ankles.

2. *Exhale*, allow your knees to fall open to the sides and place your elbows on the floor alongside your torso.

3. *Inhale*, arch the chest, press the elbows into the floor, and using that as leverage, lift the chest off the floor and arch the head back as much as is comfortable, coming to rest on the back or the top of the head. There is a huge amount of variation from one person to the next, in the degree that it is possible or safe to take the head back. You've got to use your head — both literally and figuratively. Using the neck muscles to help lift the chest is strengthening provided you don't have neck mis-

alignment or injury. You need to pay attention to your range of motion and what is possible. *This should not be practiced by anyone with neck injuries.*

4. *Exhale*, rest your fingertips at the top of your inner thighs. Keep your elbows on the floor to help support the weight of your torso. *Drishti* is straight back. Take 5 breaths.

5. *Inhale, exhale*, release the posture by gently sliding your head out, bringing your chin to your chest. Don't snap your head out of the posture, or lift it. Just slide it out, keeping the weight of the head on the floor as you bring you chin back towards your chest. Go directly to the next posture.

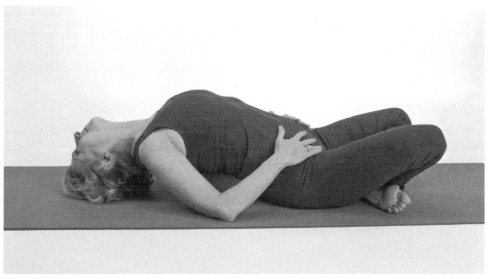

FISH POSTURE

EXTENDED LEG POSTURE

1. *Inhale*, uncross the feet and bring the knees and feet together, keeping the head in the same position

2. *Exhale*, lift the feet off the floor, and extend the legs. Stretch out the arms in front of you and bring the palms together. It is very important to tuck the tailbone and take the arch out of your lower back.

Pull the belly in and concentrate on using the abdominal muscles to hold the legs off the floor. *Drishti* is back behind you. Take 5 breaths. After your last exhalation, release the posture, bend the knees, cross your ankles, and roll up to a comfortable seated position.

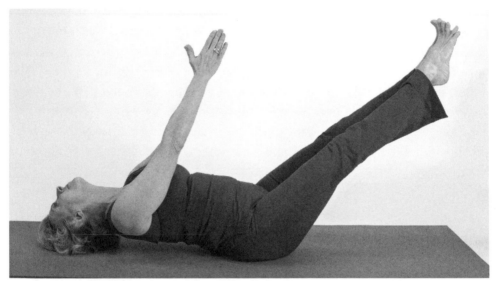

EXTENDED LEG POSTURE

BALANCING ENERGIES

Boomer Yoga is a book about waking up and paying attention. Both facets of balance — expansion and contraction — must be present in every posture, and it is up to you to find that awareness and that balance in every breath. That is why I have emphasized to such a large degree, the importance of the conscious, static contractions in each of the postures. They balance the stretch! We need to be strengthening along with stretching. The strength work creates heat and brings equilibrium between hard and soft.

FORWARD BEND EASY POSTURE

This posture is a counter pose for Fish Posture and Extended Leg Posture and reverses the backward bend of the spine that we did in the previous two postures. Clever, huh?

1. *Inhale*, come to a comfortable, cross-legged, seated position. Be aware to sit up tall, lifting the torso, yet tucking the rib cage. Cross the arms behind you and

2. *Exhale*, bend forward as far as possible. It may only be possible for you to bend slightly forward, or it may be possible for you to take your head all the way to the floor. If you need your hands on the floor in front of you to make the forward bend a bit more comfortable, that is fine. Don't allow your buttocks bones to come off the floor, which will tip you forward somewhat. *Drishti* is down past the end of your nose. Take 5 breaths. After your last exhalation, sit back up and go directly into the next posture.

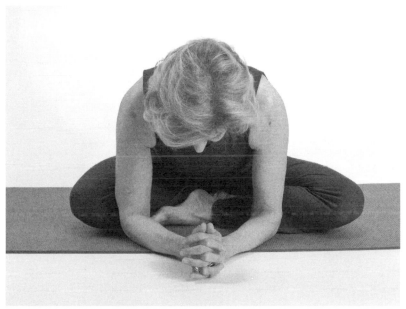

FORWARD BEND EASY POSTURE

EASY POSTURE

This is the posture that you will be using in the coming chapters (unless you choose to sit in a chair) for your breathing and meditation practices, so become familiar and comfortable with this. You are already in a comfortable cross-legged position.

1. *Inhale*, now extend your arms, and

2. *Exhale*, place the backs of your hands, or wrists or arms, on your knees with your hands open and relaxed, with the thumb and the forefinger just touching.

3. *Inhale*, lift the lower back and chest. Keep the spine long and extended, without over arching. Tuck the rib cage.

4. *Exhale*, drop the head forward a bit, moving the chin slightly towards the chest. Sit on a pillow if your knees are higher than your hips while sitting. Take 10 long and slow breaths, using very controlled *ujjayi pranayama* breathing. Make sure to check your *bandhas*. They are very important, as we go forward, to successful and correct *pranayama*. Go directly to the Lifted Easy Posture.

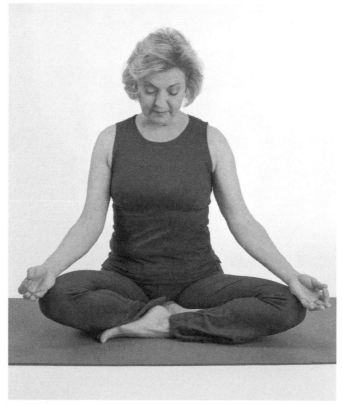

EASY POSTURE

LIFTED EASY POSTURE

1. *Inhale*, place your hands flat on the floor at your sides.

2. *Exhale*, lift yourself off the ground, pressing down into the hands, and lifting one or both of the legs. It is quite difficult and requires pretty strong abdominal muscles to lift both legs. So to begin, just push down, lean forward, and lift one leg for 5 breaths, keeping the other foot on the ground, and then switch. Take 10 breaths total, or as many as possible, increasing the number of breaths you are able to take slowly. *Drishti* is looking down as you lift and then straight out in front of you.

3. *Inhale* and *exhale*, releasing the posture. Move through a *vinyasa* as you have been doing in your practice. This is the last *vinyasa*, so go slowly and mindfully, being careful to include every cell in your body in the process. Nothing at this point should dangle outside your awareness. From Face Down Dog Posture, go directly to Relaxation Posture.

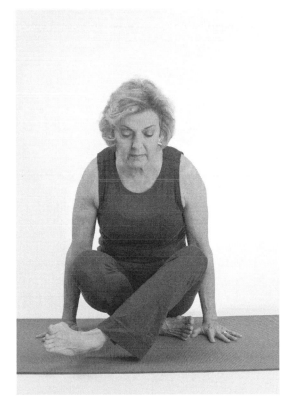

LIFTED EASY POSTURE

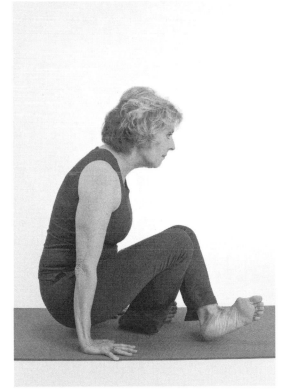

LIFTED EASY POSTURE, SIDE VIEW

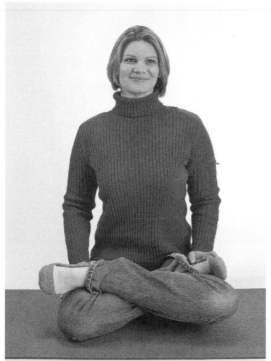

FULL LOTUS POSTURE

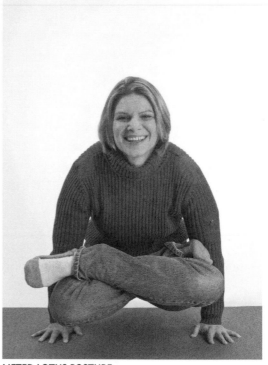

LIFTED LOTUS POSTURE

The three postures — Forward Bend Easy Posture, Easy Posture, and Lifted Easy Posture — comprise the end of your practice. They are thought to seal in all the good effects of your work. They should run together seamlessly until the last breath of the third posture. When you have limited time, you can simply do Sun Salutations and these three postures. This is thought to be minimum daily practice. These three postures are modified versions of more difficult yoga postures called Bound Lotus Posture, Lotus Posture, and Lifted Lotus Posture. They require full lotus position, which if you have the flexibility to do, you are welcome to do here instead of the Easy Posture series. Full Lotus Posture and the Lifted Lotus Posture are shown in the photographs above.

RELAXATION POSTURE

1. Lie down.

2. Come into rest position. Feet should be hip-width apart (or slightly more) and falling open to the sides. Arms at sides, palms facing up. Keep your head centered with chin level. This is an *asana*, like all the others and should be done with awareness and attention to corect alignment. It is very important here that you don't get chilled, so it is a good idea to have a light blanket or throw to cover yourself, or long-sleeve jacket or shirt handy to put on.

3. Take rest. Lie still in Relaxation Posture for at least 10 minutes. Continue to use the *ujjayi* breathing method for the first few minutes, but let it gradually fall away. Slowly allow the breath to return to normal, keeping your attention focused on the breath. Deeply let go and relax. Let the mind share the stillness and relaxation enjoyed by the body.

NOTE: If you come into rest position and you find that your lower back is a bit uncomfortable, just bring your knees to your chest and give them a hug. Hold this position for a few breaths and then roll the knees from side to side. This should alleviate any uneasiness in the lower back.

This completes the *asana* portion of the boomer yoga practice.

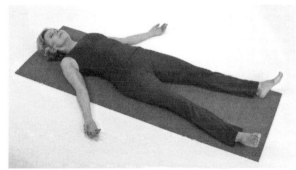

RELAXATION POSTURE

ONE MORE THING

Don't despair if you don't get all this immediately. Even with modifications and options, and as simple, balanced, and therapeutic as I have tried to make it, this *asana* routine can still be a fairly challenging practice. It will be advantageous if you can find a teacher or a video that will help you to learn the correct alignment for some of the postures. The sequence is pretty much my own invention, based on my own personal experience both as a practitioner and a teacher, so you probably won't be able to find anyone who teaches this identical sequence, unless it is someone trained by me. If it's helpful to you, you can find a listing of teachers who have been certified by me on my Web sites: www.berylbenderbirch.com or www.boomer-yoga.com. If you are just learning yoga, I cannot stress enough how important it is to go easy and take your time.

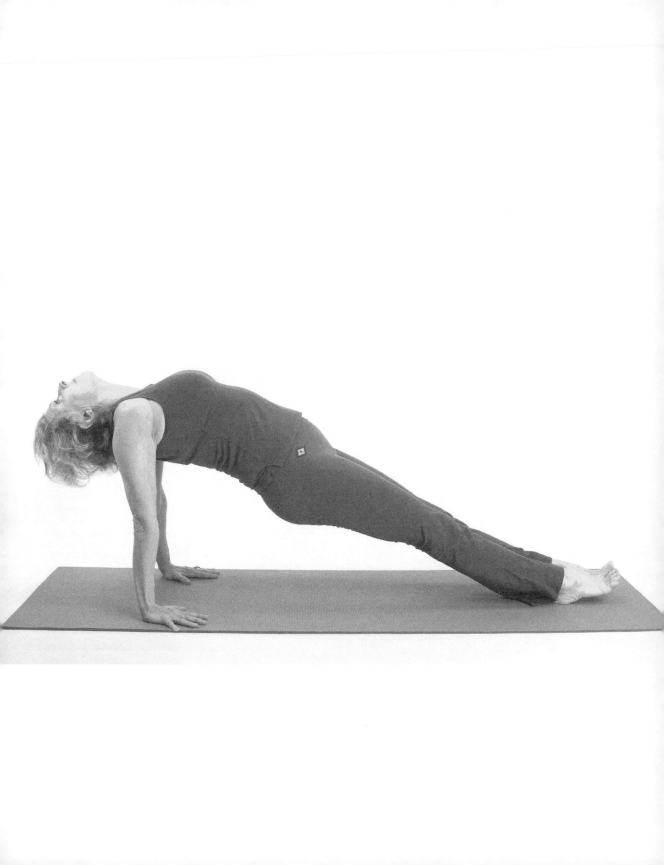

Chapter 7 CLEAR SEEING

Upping the Ante with Pranayama

Coming up on the Midtown Tunnel was like approaching a massive war zone — city police, state police, national guard troops, fire trucks, helicopters, ambulances, armed guards. Stifling and intense, the mood closed in on us. Tumbling in, half-wanting to plunge forward, and half-wanting to go back to light and sun and certainty, the few vehicles allowed into the Midtown Tunnel in New York City on Wednesday, September 12th in 2001, moved slowly toward the big, beautiful, but badly wounded city of New York. The air was dark and thick with fear and fury. The sweat rose up on everyone's brow. It was deadly silent and deafeningly loud. No one spoke. We all just prayed. No one was sure what we would find at the other end in midtown.

Although all entry in and out of the city was essentially closed down, I managed to find a way in with some friends who were rescue workers heading down to where the former World Trade Towers now lay dying as a burning, smoking, massive heap of twisted steel and rubble. I had to teach a couple of yoga classes that night and I was sure there were a lot of people who were going to be looking for refuge in a yoga class. The smoke

hadn't settled, the shock waves only now penetrating the farthest reaches of the city. There was colossal upheaval according to news reports. People were in turmoil. The city was staggering. None of us could quite get our heads around what had just happened.

As our bus emerged from the darkness into the clouded sunlight of the day, the energy of the 9/11 tragedy just crashed over us like an enormous tsunami. People wandered around the streets, lost, looking for someone to hug or to cry or just sit with. A woman sat on the curb at Thirty-ninth and Third, with her head in her hands. That picture is still imprinted in my memory. My husband Thom had been in the city. He was shaken. A Bronx Irish Catholic, he was normally ready to go to war in the event of threat or catastrophe. On the surface, not much scared him. We'd talked on the phone and he was erratic and generally freaked out. He was a long-distance runner, and on Tuesday, when everyone else was running north in the city, away from downtown, he was running south, towards Wall Street to see what he could do to help. One of our yoga students, our good friend, Pat Brown, was a highly decorated captain in the New York City Fire Department. We knew he'd been one of the first firemen into the towers and we were both pretty sure he had been in the towers when they fell.

There was an enormous feeling of connectedness, a huge family, suffering a great loss and coming together to grieve, wail, support one another and wonder what was going to happen next. Strangers hugged each other and shared seats and cabs and glasses of wine. Everyone was in shock and on edge. What in the hell had just happened? This is New York city. Those buildings were the World Trade Towers, for God's sake. We were stunned into silence. Enormous clouds of debris-filled smoke and ash blanketed the lower part of the city. You could smell the death and devastation. We all knew, by that point, that thousands had been killed in the disaster.

Over the next few days, the information started to filter out, about which floors in the towers were hit the hardest. Thom and I had a bunch of students who lived on the Upper East Side, where we taught classes, but who worked downtown. I knew that a couple of regular students worked for Marsh & McLennan, another for Cantor Fitzgerald, two of the corporations headquartered on the floors of the towers that were hit directly. I had the ominous sense of knowing that at least a few of my students, besides Pat, had to have been killed. That was the thing we all realized as the weeks went by — everyone (and not just in the city, but for miles around stretching in every direction) knew someone who had not turned up at home or a friend's home or was still missing. We all — the

entire Northeast, the entire country practically — fearfully waited for the news that our friend or family member or spouse or student or associate or neighbor had been killed.

Yoga classes that night were filled with fear and prayer, tears and trembling. People came, not knowing where else to go or what else to do. They walked in, weakened, with heads hanging low, panting, stunned, stumbling around and feeling faint. One woman came with her feet blistered and bloodied after running from her office on Fulton Street and Broadway to escape the burgeoning clouds of debris that mushroomed out in every direction when the towers fell, then, after taking off her high heels, she walked barefoot five or six miles to her uptown home on Ninety-second Street. I hugged everyone who came in to class. We cried. There were no words.

We did a little bit of *asana*, slowly breathing and moving, but people were collapsing — kneeling, bent over with chest to knees, head to floor. The movement helped to ease the tension, and the work of focusing on the breath brought us for an instant, a moment, out of the penetrating visual memories of what we had experienced to a nanosecond of emptiness and relief. Whether running from the collapsing wreckage or helplessly empathizing with our brothers and sisters via television, collectively we desperately wanted to relieve the intense pressure, the wringing tension, to empty our minds.

I gathered everyone in a circle, lit some candles, and we sat together and breathed. I led people through a few rounds of the very same *ujjayi* breathing that you have been using all through your work with this book. However, instead of being combined with *asana*, we used it as a stand-alone practice. What we actually did is called *sama vritti ujjayi pranayama*, or "equal" (*sama*) "movement" (*vritti*) *ujjayi pranayama*. It is the way that *ujjayi* should be practiced and emphasizes not just concentration on the sound of the breath, but concentration on making the inhalation and the exhalation exactly equal — in sound, depth, length, and so forth, although it takes some time to get the hang of the balance between the in-breath and the out-breath. Follow the breath, listen to the breath, bring your attention to the breath. Close your mouth and just breathe. That's all.

FINDING RELIEF

Since you have been doing this practice for some time by now, I'm sure you can relate to the power of the *ujjayi* breathing. Haven't you used this breathing technique many times on its own, outside of yoga class, other than in combination with your *asana* practice?

What is it about the technique that makes it so powerful? Why is it so effective in helping us to relax or get grounded and centered? Well, for one thing, it requires our attention. It doesn't happen by itself. Focusing on this breath, which is what it takes in order to *do* it, brings our attention to the *now*. The breath is always in the present moment and for as long as we can focus on it, we are here — not in the past, not in the future, but now. So,

if for an instant, we can be with the breath, then we cannot be plastered up against our thoughts of yesterday's disaster, no matter how catastrophic. Nor can we be trembling with thoughts of what might happen to us tomorrow. For that instant we are free of attachment to the past or future. We are free of anger, hatred, and fear.

This was certainly one of the times in my life, and the life of many others as well, when being present and leaning into "what is" was excruciatingly difficult. Some things change us slightly, or for a short time — some things change us forever. This was one of those events that changed us and our world quickly, dramatically, and irreversibly. People sought escape — as we do so often when we are in pain — in many different ways and via many different avenues. People got drunk, got laid, they plunged into rescue work and community service, they divorced, got married, quit their jobs, and moved to the country. Others came to New York to help pick up the pieces. Others came to yoga class.

The days went by in a fog. It was hard to do anything but watch the television. No matter what else one needed to do, if it wasn't related to rescue or volunteer work, it seemed irrelevant. I walked downtown on Saturday or Sunday, and I clearly remember the Chelsea Jean store on John Street and Broadway. The windows were blown out and racks of Levis were covered with rubble and ash. Chase Manhattan Bank, at Fulton and Broadway, looked like a combat zone. The windows were gone and the whole bank was littered with debris, dust, ash, computers, desks, phones, photos. Depressed workers were beginning to vacuum. It seemed so futile. The mess downtown was overwhelming. Where to even start to clean up? We made sandwiches and offered food and shelter to those who were evacuated from their buildings. We stood in line to donate blood. Volunteers kept coming to the city.

My friend, JoAnn Difede, a research psychologist and director of the Post Traumatic Stress Disorder (PSTD) Clinic, at the time a little known program at Weill Cornell Medical Center on the Upper East Side of New York, called to see if I might be available to help out with the families of burn victims that had been evacuated or escaped from the towers. JoAnn and I were familiar with one another's work, and she wanted someone with fairly extensive professional experience in the field of yoga to come in and offer some assistance to the people flooding her offices.

Before 9/11, I don't think too many people outside the medical community were familiar with PTSD. But suddenly Dr. Difede was at the center of an enormous national demand for treatment for firemen, policemen, families of those who had perished or were missing, city workers, government workers, employees of corporations who had been affected, and anyone else who had escaped from downtown that beautifully sunny and clear Tuesday morning. The media called her non-stop for quotes and explanations of what people were feeling, network news called for interviews, hospitals around the country, looking to treat traumatized Americans, called for advice, and unexpectedly JoAnn was the go-to person for expert advice on PTSD.

When I phoned her back, it took me awhile to get through. She had several staff members working to assist with fielding phone calls, scheduling, and organizing requests for help.

"JoAnn? It's Beryl. How are you?"

"Oh my God, it's beyond description."

"How are you managing?"

"Oh, I'm okay. But people are freaked out — understandably. There is so much work to do. I've gotta go. Can you come in and work with the families of the burn victims here at the Burn Center at Weill Medical?"

"Oh my God, Jo Ann, I don't know. What could I possibly do to help? Teach them yoga?"

"Isn't there something you could do? Just help them to sleep, or have a moment of freedom from their overwhelming grief. Have them breath or meditate or something? When can you come? Tomorrow?"

"Well, okay."

"Come at 2:00 — meet me at my office. Bye."

Wow. My mind was spinning. What in the world would I do? I'd never done anything like this before. What could I say that would help? These were families whose loved ones had been horrendously burned in the fires and explosions, many of them on more than 80 percent of their bodies and their chances of survival were minimal. What do you say to family members who are praying for a miracle but fearing the worst? What can you do to comfort them?

When I walked into a small room on the same floor in the hospital as the Burn Center, I was nervous. It was filled with comfortable couches and chairs, a table, and just a few men and women — relatives of people in nearby rooms who were wrapped in bandages from head to toe and heavily medicated for relief from unbelievable pain, many dying, others struggling for life — the mothers, fathers, daughters, sons, husbands, and wives sat stunned and silent.

They all looked up as I came into the room, waiting for news on someone, somewhere. They looked exhausted. As it turned out, none of them had slept in nearly a week — since the towers crashed. I didn't assume anything. I didn't assume I could help. I didn't assume I knew anything that could be of use. Faced with such incredible suffering, how could anyone go on with what now seemed to be the completely mundane activities of life without falling into total despair? There was such a sense of hopelessness in the room. I didn't think that Jesus Christ or Buddha or Mother Theresa could have done much in this situation, what could I do? I knew I couldn't just walk in there and carry on like I had some secret formula that would erase their suffering. I just sat down quietly at the table and put my head in my hands. "Dear Lord," I thought, "give me strength and the right words to say." Someone came over and put his hand on my shoulder. We both

started to cry. That was sort of it — the ice breaker.

I remembered what I did in yoga class earlier in the week, sitting with everyone and breathing — all of us together. It was the breathing that seemed to have offered the most relief and the most comfort. I introduced myself and suggested that we, all together, see if there was something we could discover, something we could do, that would help us all to sleep, to deal with the tragedy, to grieve but to avoid despair and depression. "Let's just sit," I suggested. I moved everyone into a circle and had them close their eyes. And what happened after that — I don't remember so well, except I slowly came around to teaching them *ujjayi* breathing. Breathe in, breathe out, with sound. That's all. Get the sound and pay attention to it, and see if you can make the inhalation and the exhalation the same length and make them sound as much alike as possible.

Within minutes, everyone at the table was making the slow, controlled, aspirant sound of the inhalation and sibilant sound of the exhalation of the *ujjayi* breath. They just *got* it. They hung on it as a life line. The time became timeless. We sat like that for nearly thirty or forty minutes, but no one had a clue how long we had been there. I kept an eye on them. Each of them just climbed into the breath and went away to a place that was quiet and peaceful — for a moment. One man fell asleep during the session, God bless him. It was joyful to see him sleeping. Another woman actually smiled and came and hugged me. I don't know, I can't say it was some miraculous cure for suffering, but it did help. This was not an easy time. I said to the group, "I hope you will remember that well enough to use in your most difficult moments — it will help you to sleep and to find strength. Thank you. I'll be back tomorrow."

The work with the families went so well that Dr. Difede suggested I return to the hospital the next day and work with some of the burn victims themselves, which I was now eager to do. The nervousness was gone and all I could think of was, "What can I do to help?" Funny, when you stop worrying about how you will perform and just focus on helping to reduce suffering, somehow the Universe gives you inspiration and you find the right words and the right action. One man I sat and breathed with for many days was, ironically, from India. He was especially taken with the *ujjayi* breathing and every day when we finished, he would ask if I could return the following day. Perhaps he felt some ancient, genetic connection to this yogic breathing technique.

Well, in the long run, the program was so well received that it became a model program for using yoga therapy for pain and stress management. Dr. Difede was so impressed with the positive results that she had me teach *ujjayi* breathing to her staff, who, in turn, taught it to their patients. Months later, she applied for a grant from the Greater New York Hospital Association, who then funded a program for yoga classes and training in *ujjayi* breathing for the medical center and hospital employees. I initially taught the course then passed it over to a number of my teachers. Now, years later, the program is still growing and bringing much-needed stress-relief to the employees at Weill Cornell Medical Center.

ENERGY MANAGEMENT

Occasionally, you might see *pranayama* defined as "breathing exercises." Well, we do carry out breathing routines for our *pranayama* practice, but the true meaning is a great deal more refined than simply huffing and puffing in and out. The word *pranayama* is composed of two words: *prana*, which means "life force" or "energy," or when used in the word *pranayama* it can mean "breath;" and *ayama*, which means "extension" or "stretch." So literally translated, *pranayama* generally means "breath extension" or "energy extension." If we look at *pranayama* as an important form of *tapas*, or as a way to burn impurities and make room for *prana*, then this is a pretty suitable definition. When we practice *pranayama*, we are actually expanding our ability to hold *prana*. However, we can look at the definition in another way, as composed of the two words *prana* and *yama*. The word *yama* means "restraint" or the opposite of *ayama*. This changes the definition of *pranayama* from a practice of expansion to one of restraint or pulling in. This seems like a very different explanation. Holding energy back is the opposite of stretching energy. Now, how can that be? So which is it?

I have come to realize over the years that it is

both. In order to expand our energy, we need to learn to control it, to manage it. Don't you find that true in everyday life? Eventually, we begin to realize that the more careful we are about to whom and to what we give our attention, our *energy*, the more *energy* we seem to have available to be able to give. This process of discernment is called *viveka* in yoga. Mindful breathing requires that we *stretch* to gain control over the breath, and as we do we are developing our ability to manage our energy. Haven't you noticed that already in your practice? As we enlarge our capacity to take in *prana*, we increase our capacity to put it to more efficient and effective use — we manage it better! Where our *attention* goes, our *prana* follows.

Once we have learned to use the *ujjayi pranayama* in our *asana* practice, we can begin to use it on its own as a form of mindfulness training and stress reduction and preparation for meditation. For those times when we cannot do *asana* or want to add to our *asana* practice and move deeper into the yoga methodology, we can begin to work with mindful breathing. *Pranayama* is the fourth limb of classical yoga. It follows *asana*, the third limb, with the intention being that we need to first get our bones and muscles organized with *asana*, the most basic, tangible part of the system. Then we can move on to more subtle levels of practice like *pranayama*. Since *pranayama* is about working with the breath, it requires that we have the ability to actually focus on the breath. In order to actually *do pranayama* we need to be able to sit comfortably, without fidgeting, and then bring our attention to our breathing. If we are still quite stiff and tight, or in physical pain when we try to sit for *pranayama* practice, then focusing on the breath will not only be difficult, it will be impossible.

There are many types and forms of *pranayama* — which include retentions, alternate nostril breathing, abdominal pumping, and so forth. The purpose of them all is pretty much

MOVING ENERGY

Remember, in the practice of *pranayama* we are actually trying to move, or direct, *prana*. This ability to move *prana* in the physical or energetic body is called *prana dharana* or "energy concentration." Because it is easier to simply follow the breath with our attention we need to be able to do that first before we can actually move energy around in our body. If we can't follow the breath, we can't move *prana*. Although this may sound specious, it is all very logical, and follows a strict set of instructions, as set down in *The Yoga Sutra* two thousand years ago. Amazingly enough, these instructions are still relevant today. So we practice for hours, days, weeks, and months, just concentrating on the breath, and slowly we begin to understand what is meant by actually *moving* energy. Think of what a handy skill it might be to have, if and when you need it — and we will all need it sooner or later.

to continue the work of *asana* — which is to further develop mindfulness and to deepen detoxification. The various techniques of different schools and traditions can become fairly intricate and complicated. However, what is important to remember is that the point of the increasing complexity is to train the mind, using more challenging assignments to stay focused over longer periods of time.

Since we are already familiar with the *ujjayi* method of *pranayama*, and because it is a very effective and powerful technique, we are going to continue to use it for our *pranayama* practice. As you become comfortable with simply sitting and breathing, we will add some small pauses, or retentions, called *kumbhaka* in yoga, in between the breaths. The objective of using short retentions is simply to intensify our concentration and to strengthen and amplify the power of the breath and the *prana* it carries.

The great thing about understanding how to use *pranayama* on its own is that in those times when we are ill or injured or not in a place or position to do *asana*, we can still do our yoga.

Because anything can change, disappear, transform in an instant, we look to our *pranayama* practice to help us deal with the overwhelming instability of our world. One breath at a time. And what does that teach us? It teaches us to be present and grateful and content with this moment — because we don't really know what could happen in the next moment.

THE FIRST LIMB OF YOGA

In Book 2 of *The Yoga Sutra*, which is the very practical portion of *The Yoga Sutra*, following the very esoteric Book 1, Patanjali delineates the eight-limbed methodology of classical yoga. He starts out by giving an explanation of the first two limbs, the five *yamas* and the five *niyamas*. The *yamas* are the moral preliminaries and practices that are set down as general guidelines for right conduct. These are *ahmisa* (non-violence), *satya* (truth), *asteya* (non-stealing), *aparigraha* (non-greediness or non-accumulation) and, *bramacharya* (moderation). Patanjali calls them the *maha-vratum*, or the Great Vows, and says that they are not limited by "class, place, time, or circumstance." In other words, they apply to all those who wish to practice yoga, at all times, regardless of religion, culture, nationality, social or economic status, or individual circumstances.

According to yoga thought, the *yamas* are the root of our spiritual evolutionary process, and we really can't begin to transform or evolve until we have some understanding of these five principles. They are the fundamentals of the entire yoga discipline and the ethical foundation on which everything else is built. You can say you are *doing yoga*; you can wear nice stylish yoga clothes, read yoga books, go to classes, and even, go to India. But until you spend a little time thinking about the *yamas* and the role they play in your life, you are a long way from the true practice of yoga. The interesting thing about them, and the *niyamas* as well, is that even though they are limb one and limb two of the classical yoga path, most people who say they are *doing yoga* (*asana*) not only don't think about these first two limbs, but don't even know about them until well into years of working with *asana*, which is why I am only bringing them up now. As I've said throughout the book, most people begin their study of yoga with the practice of *asana*, and that generally takes all their attention for quite awhile. Because we often have a specific need that we hope yoga will address, we become wrapped up in focusing on the physical portion of the practice. But as a person spends more and more time going to classes, and perhaps moves from classes at a gym or health club to classes at a yoga studio, he or she will begin to be exposed to more and more of the yoga philosophy and lifestyle that accompanies the *exercise* portion.

So how do you do the *yamas*? Granted, these five principles are huge topics. And you might even think, well, if the *yamas* are the first limb and *asana* is the third limb of classical yoga, does this mean I have to practice perfect truth, for example, in order to go on to *asana*? How could that even be possible? Nobody practices *perfect satya* (truth). Or *perfect ahimsa* (non-violence) for that matter. In fact, if we are in body, which it's pretty safe to assume we all are, then perfect *ahimsa* is impossible. Every time we take a step, we are killing some little thing — some worm, some insect, some bacteria. So what do we do?

Well, first we make an effort to understand these five principles and how they might

THE EIGHT LIMBS OF CLASSICAL (*ASTANGA*) YOGA

1. *Yama* (restraint)

   There are five *yamas*: *ahimsa* (non-violence), *satya* (truth), *asteya* (non-stealing), *aparigraha* (non-greediness, or non-accumulation), and *brahmacharya* (to walk with God, often translated as "moderation")

2. *Niyama* (observance)

   There are five *niyamas*: *saucha* (purity, cleanliness), *santosha* (contentment), *tapas* (to burn), *svadhaya* (self-study, study of the scriptures), and *Isvara pranidhana* (surrender to God)

3. *Asana* (postures)

4. *Pranayama* (restraint of the *prana*, breathing control)

5. *Pratyahara* (turning in of the senses)

6. *Dharana* (concentration)

7. *Dhyana* (meditation)

8. *Samadhi* (bliss, the Enlightened State)

guide our actions. We contemplate their meanings. Really. We sit down and ask ourselves questions like, do I tell the truth? Can I watch myself to see how much of the time I don't tell the truth in order to protect myself or because I feel inadequate or to impress someone. Am I non-violent? Am I compassionate? Do I recognize that all sentient creatures love life? Do I care about animal suffering, for example? Or do I just care about myself, my family, and my tribe?

Watch anything, birds, insects, fish — they all move towards life and away from something that might represent a threat to life. How mindful am I that human life isn't any more or less sacred than any other form of life? Now that takes a great deal of consciousness and awareness to "get."

Do we steal? Well, of course not, you might respond. But do you "steal" other people's ideas, and claim them as your own? Do you steal time from others? Are you greedy? That's a great one to play around with. We are all greedy in various ways. How much stuff have we accumulated? Have we realized, that our "stuff" isn't bringing all that much satisfaction and that *nothing in the world of form* will ever bring lasting happiness?

THE SECOND LIMB OF CLASSICAL YOGA

The five *niyamas* are a little more practical than the *yamas*. They are like five substantial stepping stones that offer a tangible way out of the mud, through the impenetrable forest,

and into the light. We are going to look at the first two *niyamas*: *saucha* (purity) and *santosha* (contentment) in this chapter, and we'll save the last three for chapter 10. *Saucha* and *santosha* are easy to understand and pretty easy to put into play.

Saucha refers to keeping the body clean and pure, bathing carefully and wearing clean clothes, and nourishing the body with life-supporting foods. I like to add, in my teacher training courses, that it includes using dental floss. Being aware of *saucha* and developing it as habit is a little easier than adopting *ahimsa* (non-violence) or *satya* (truth) completely into our lives. It's easy to actually do, because it involves something concrete and tangible. We can bathe. We can keep our clothes clean. But *saucha* also refers to mental purity and asks that we work to keep our mind free of negative and polluted thoughts. Here it kind of runs into *ahimsa* and *satya* a bit. Working to not think negative thoughts isn't that different from not having violent or untruthful thoughts. The *niyamas*, like the limbs themselves, all run into one another. They are not like separate radio stations, where you just tune in 88.3 on your dial and listen only to one frequency. They flow together, influencing and directing the progress and course of one another.

Santosha means to enjoy and accept what is and to be grateful for what we have. It means to accept and be content with this moment, instead of being in resistance to what is. But suppose "what is" is unbearable? Suppose we are stuck in the mud? Or stuck in a horrible

UNDERSTANDING THE *YAMAS*

I have observed that as people begin the practice of yoga, they begin to be aware of the ways in which the various *yamas* manifest in their daily lives. People make an effort to be more truthful, accumulate less, take only what is offered, walk a little closer to the middle path, and be kinder. It just sort of comes along with the territory. For example, you can't *try* to be compassionate — compassion develops as a result of increasing awareness and through accessing deeper levels of consciousness. And how do we become more aware? Well, that is what this entire book is about. We quiet the noise of the mind, through learning to focus on the present, and as a result, the fog lifts and we see a little more clearly.

job or relationship? Or in a war or economic meltdown? How can we be content with that? Contentment with this moment doesn't mean that you accept every injustice or abuse that comes along or that nothing ever changes. It simply means that "for this moment" you find gratitude for something — a job, a friend, a healthy body, or even your life or your awareness. You think to yourself, "Okay, this sucks, but I have created this. No one has done this to me. God doesn't 'hate' me and love everyone else. Let me see what I can do to move out of this situation." And you say "thank you" to no one in particular, just thank you. And you cultivate gratitude. And, again, because you are making an effort to practice, clarity comes. Something changes. Shift happens.

WHERE THE MIND GOES, *PRANA* FOLLOWS

In yoga it is believed that our "bodies" are comprised of "five sheaths," or what in Sanskrit is called, *pancha kosha*. The most basic sheath is the *anna-maya-kosha* or the "sheath composed of food." The next sheath, more subtle, is the *prana-maya-kosha*, or the "sheath composed of life force," or *prana*. It is in this layer, or sheath, that the energy of *prana* flows. It travels through channels, or *nadis*, and it is our practice of *pranayama* that helps to clear the *nadis* for smooth-flowing *prana* and teaches us how to consciously direct and control this flow. The detox work of *asana* clears and cleans out the "food" sheath and prepares us for work in the *prana* sheath. But before it is possible to condense and direct *prana* toward a certain objective, it helps to understand what *prana* is, and whether or not there is enough of the stuff in your body to do anything with it. As we learn to pay attention, we can *feel* if and when we are *prana*-deficient, or conversely, *prana*-rich.

The yogis say that when we are disturbed, our *prana* is scattered. The more disturbed we are, the more our life force is decimated

PLUGGING THE LEAKS

In your *asana* training, you begin to specifically notice where you are tight or weak, where you get distracted and by what, where the breath is shallow, and when you are impatient or uncomfortable. You learn to pay attention to when you get distracted, or go "off." And when you notice you are distracted, this is what I call noticing an "energy leak" — the *prana* is going off into space somewhere on a stream of thought forms (where the mind goes, *prana* follows). So what do you do? You bring yourself back to the present moment. That process of bringing yourself back to the present moment and refocusing your attention is the primary technique for unplugging from something that is taking your attention, or your *prana*.

and lost. To be strong and healthy we need to learn to keep *prana* inside our body. Thus, we learn not only to spot leaks, but also how to clean out the body so it can hold more *prana*. If we are filled with toxins and clogged or injured body parts, how will we find room to store *prana*? Do we know what it is we do that actually wastes our *prana*? If we run around, trying to get things done, but nothing gets accomplished, then we know we are going to feel tired and as if we wasted time and energy. That's pretty clear.

But what about all the thousands and thousands of drains on our energy reserves that are more subtle, drains that originate in our mind — worry, anxiety, anger, nervousness, and so forth? Can we see that worrying about something that may or may not happen in the future can cost us energy in the present?

As our yoga practice becomes more advanced and fluid, we begin to develop a sense of what spiritual teachers and teachings refer to as being the "Witness," or the "Observer." This is the ability to step outside yourself and

observe your thoughts, your feelings, your emotions, rather than just identifying with them. For most of us, for a good portion of our lives, who we are at any moment is totally determined by what we are thinking or feeling. There is no space between our thoughts and who we think we are. We are our thoughts. I always refer to that in my teachings as being "plastered up against conditioned thought," like wallpaper on a wall. Splat. No space between the two.

But slowly, as we practice being mindful, we begin to see that we can "choose" to either be what a particular thought is dictating, or we can separate from the thought, and simply observe it. Yoga becomes, for us, an objective perceptual system that helps us to identify when, where, and how we are losing our *prana*, or in other words, how we are getting caught up with thoughts that direct us to a past argument with our sister, or an insult from a co-worker, or an abuse by a family member, or to fears or anxieties about the future, all of which are costing us *prana*.

Often, when we begin the practice of yoga, it may seem that we are in the darkest hour before the dawn. The practice of the postures can be awkward and difficult. This is not fun. We may wonder if we are ever going to see the light. But somehow, we persevere, and one day, seemingly out of the blue, a ray of light begins to show itself. We start to see that this practice we are undertaking is beginning to change us slightly. We have been doing the *asana* routine and it's not quite as unpleasant as it may have been when we started. We are opening up a little bit. We are developing a little more strength. We have dug up a few spots where our *prana* was blocked, or we discovered a few things we were giving our energy to that needed to be let go of. Some of the stiffness starts to move, which may have seemed impossible when we started. This is the first glimmer of conscious evolution.

GETTING SETTLED

There is no way you can actually do this *pranayama* practice and read the details that follow about how to do it at the same time. The best that might happen is that you can read through this, making mental notes, and then sit and try to recreate a "tape of instructions" in your mind. (It might be helpful for you to know that there is a companion CD available from my Web sites, www.berylbenderbirch.com and www.boomer-yoga.com, which will guide you through the practice, and help you to learn how, in due course, to practice on your own.)

Take a moment now to do whatever is necessary to prepare your space for your *pranayama* practice and to minimize any possible distractions. This might mean closing a door, opening a window, posting a "do not disturb for 30 minutes" sign on the door, lighting a candle, or turning out the lights. Then settle yourself down.

Sit comfortably. Make sure you will be comfy and warm enough while you sit, either by wrapping a shawl around your shoulders or a blanket over your legs. You are welcome to sit in a chair or cross-legged on the floor on a pillow. If you are unable to sit, then you can lie down, with a flat pillow under your head. You can pretty much only be at ease sitting on the floor if your knees are lower than your hips when you sit, so sitting with a pillow under your buttocks elevates your hips and makes sitting easier. If you are sitting in a chair, don't lean back or rest against the back of your chair. Sit with your back straight with both feet flat on the floor. Drop the chin slightly. Now, close your eyes and rest your hands, folding them in your lap or placing them on your knees.

Notice any physical discomfort that might be taking your attention. Just watch for a minute, what is calling out for your attention? Your knee or hip or back? See if you can lessen the uneasiness with a slight shift in position.

Now get comfortable again and continue to watch. At some point you will need to settle in and come to stillness. If this is totally impossible, you might need to postpone *pranayama* work and go back to doing a bit more *asana* until sitting with stillness becomes easier. It doesn't take long to see that this sitting business can be physically and mentally challenging — which is why *asana* precedes *pranayama* in the eight-limbed path of classical yoga! We actually do the *asana* practice to get the body healthy, open, strong, and flexible enough and the mind trained well enough in preliminary concentration, to sit comfortably and quietly for breath work and, eventually, meditation.

PREPARING FOR THE ACTUAL PRANAYAMA PRACTICE

Once you have physically settled in, bring your attention to the surrounding environment. What are you picking up? What is going on? Noise? Can you hear anything? Wind? Voices? Traffic passing? Rain falling? Observe for a few moments. Listen objectively. Try not to judge the sounds as good sounds or bad sounds. Just let them be as they are — neutral. Accept them as part of what *is* for this moment.

See if you can develop a sense of where you are. Place yourself in space, surrounded by a 360-degree awareness. Sit with that for a moment or two.

Now see if you can turn your attention inward and listen to the inner environment. What thoughts are filling your awareness? Are you bored? Restless? Waiting for whatever it is that will come next? Take a couple of moments to just observe what is going on? Are you re-running an event that took place earlier in the day that got stuck in your mind somehow? Notice who or what is taking your attention. Are you thinking of something to eat? To do? See if you can step back and just sit and observe what is coming up on the screen of your mind. Whatever you notice — let it bubble up, like oxygen bubbles from the bottom of a lake. Don't suppress your thoughts — simply watch them. And let them drift by like clouds in the sky.

After you practice watching your thoughts for a bit, slowly bring your attention to your breathing, your normal, natural breathing. Ahhhhhhhh, the breathing? Did we even notice our breathing until this moment? What is going on with the breath? See if you can just watch your breath without changing it. This, of course, is impossible to do because the moment we observe anything, it changes it slightly. But see if you can just watch, without doing anything with your breath. Don't make it slower, don't use *ujjayi* — not yet anyway — just watch your normal breathing.

Let's see if we can make some detailed observations about the breath. You cannot do this while you are reading, so see if you can just develop a sense of the various qualities of your breath that we are going to view. Is the breath high or low in the body? Take a moment to really observe this quality until you have an answer in your mind. Then go on. Is it dry or humid? Slow or rapid? Deep or shallow? Labored or effortless? Warm or cool? Sit and watch your breath as you might observe a beautiful animal, or an interesting person who captured your attention.

SETTING SAIL

Next, slowly begin to put *ujjayi* breathing in place. Observe the differences between just your natural breathing and, now, your controlled *ujjayi* breathing. This is *ujjayi pranayama*. It must be supported by *mula* and *uddiyana bandha*. Without the locks, the *prana*, or *apana* (as this form of *prana* is called in the lower part of the abdomen), will simply drain out, like water in a bathtub that you have forgotten to plug! The water runs and runs, but the tub never fills, because as fast as the water runs in, it runs out.

So, make sure through all of this that you continuously give a small portion of your awareness, your *prana*, to keeping *mula bandha* and *uddiyana bandha* in place. You know where the 1st *chakra* is at the perineum. Just send a little energy there and make sure that, not only is the gateway to the *chakra* closed, but that it is locked. You know where the 2nd *chakra* is, just a couple of inches below the navel. Send a little of your awareness there and make sure that that gate, that energy center, stays locked. I like to imagine that I have posted a little sentry at each of the *chakras*, and it is their job to make sure the gates remain locked.

Take the next few moments to simply attempt to stay focused on your *ujjayi* breathing. It should feel like listening to an old friend, pleasant, familiar, and relaxed. Now, to up the ante a bit, see if you can make the in-breath and the out-breath, *sama vritti*, of "equal movement." That will take attention — as you listen closely, make an effort to make each half of a complete breath equal to the other in length, and depth (or height), and sound. Spend some time developing a rhythm that is comfortable for you — not too fast and not too slow. This isn't a contest. You aren't trying to see how slowly you can breathe. You are trying to train your mind to pay attention to the breath. Working with *sama vritti* is a wonderful exercise and takes full attention. However, after a few minutes the mind will get bored with this exercise as well. At first it is engaging, but eventually, the mind decides it doesn't like all this focus and discipline and it wanders off in search of some excitement. Every time you realize that you have lost your focus, and the mind has kicked in and started thinking, just notice the thought, and bring your attention back to your breath. Inhale and exhale. Inhale and exhale.

ADDING RETENTION

Now we are going to add one more element to our practice. After each breath, both the inhalation and the exhalation, you are going to simply add a short pause. This is called a *kumbhaka*, or "retention." You will just hold the inhale or the exhale for a beat, a second, and then continue. This will, for a short time, add a little excitement for your mind, but before long the mind will begin to get bored again and be off and running. The mind hates to be disciplined and will wander off again and again. The mind will get fed up. The body will clamor for your attention. Let that be okay. Let that pass, like clouds drifting by on a windy day. Refocus, again with patience and perseverance, like you were patiently teaching a dog to sit. You tell your dog to sit. The dog sits. Then the dog gets up and walks off. You bring the dog back and again, you say, "Sit." The dog sits for a moment and then sees a bird and jumps up and chases it. You try again. It is the same with the mind. Eventually, the dog learns to sit and stay (except maybe Siberian huskies). Eventually, our mind learns to be still.

If you are using my CD, you will hear me asking throughout, "Where is your attention now?" If you are not using the CD, you will need to do that for yourself. Catch yourself. Notice the minute your mind moseys off. Sometimes the mind will launch a movie. Our attention gets caught up with the movie and it takes some time before we realize that we have lost our focus and are totally involved in the movie. We have walked out of the room, down the street, off with one of friends, and we are shopping at Target, and then suddenly we notice that the mind has taken us out, and off and away. Every time your mind is distracting you by "thinking" again (and again and again — whew!), bring the attention back. Listen to the sound. Let each breath carry you deeper into the center of your Self. Relax, melt into each breath. Allow the mind to quiet — falling deeply into the stillness.

When the body first begins to claim your attention, perhaps your back or your knee starts to bother you, or you feel anxious for freedom from regulating your breath, there is a strong desire on the part of the mind for this training to be O-V-E-R! The first few times this happens, see if you can mentally just send energy to that place that is claiming your attention. See if you can dissipate the discomfort without moving and try to stay focused. If, eventually, the discomfort becomes overwhelming, go ahead and adjust and reposition yourself slightly and bring your attention back to the breath, always supporting the *pranayama* with the *bandhas*.

At some point, after weeks and months of practice, you may begin to have the sensation of actual energy, or *prana*, more than just the breath, circulating around your body — maybe in the body, maybe just outside the body. This sounds a little *out there*, but it happens. If you practice long enough, you will feel it. This is *prana* moving. At this point, you can experiment. Try sending the *prana* to a specific place in your body. Then see if you can actually feel any change in that part of your body. Do this from time to time and see what happens. Once you can feel this happening, you can begin to expand your ability to actually move *prana* to more general and/or remote conditions or locations. Visualize sending *prana* to a condition that needs healing, whether in your body or in your life. Or send *prana* to a friend who is suffering and needs help. This is a wonderful practice, but should be done at the end of your practice, because it no longer focuses your attention on your breath, but takes you out into the world of conditions and circumstances. It's okay and good work, but you should realize that it is no longer the *pranayama* practice, but a form of visualization and sending energy. Be sure to spend quite a bit of time mastering your skill in *pranayama* before you begin distracting yourself with the challenging but tremendously important tasks of healing yourself — and the world.

To end your *pranayama* practice, begin to deepen your breath and very gently start your return journey to waking consciousness. Take a long full breath and draw it out. You may feel like stretching. Keep the eyes closed. Reach to your right knee with your left hand, take a big inhale, then exhale and twist to your right. Release, then inhale again, and reach to your left knee with your right hand. Exhale and twist to your left. Release, and then place your hands on the floor or behind you on the seat of the chair. Inhale and then exhale and arch back. Release and then place your hands on your knees or on the floor in front of you and inhale, then exhale, and curl forward, rounding your back. Then come back to sitting straight, and with your eyes still closed, rub your hands together until you feel some heat in your hands. Rest your eyes, covering them with the palms of your hands. Then,

slowly, begin to move the hands away from your eyes and back to your lap as you slowly begin to open your eyes, allowing the light back in, and the sense of sight to re-emerge. Take a deep breath. Feel refreshed, relaxed, and at the center of your Self.

Take time to sit quietly and try to practice this breathing technique every day. If that's not possible, then try to do some *pranayama* at least three to four times per week. Or whenever, you feel like you need to recharge or de-stress or reconnect with your Self. This work, if it interests you, is preparing you for the more advanced aspects of your yoga practice. *Pranayama* is the beginning, after *asana*, of developing concentration and learning the skill of the fifth limb *pratyahara*, which is the turning inward of the senses. Don't get frazzed over this. It's a whole, long journey and is why the yoga methodology is called a "path." After weeks and months and years of regular practice, you may actually begin to shift your awareness from the four outer limbs of yoga (*yama, niyama, asana, pranayama*) across the bridge of the fifth limb (*pratyahara*) to the three inner limbs (*dharana, dhyana,* and *samadhi*), and have the experience of real *dharana* (concentration) or *dhyana* (meditation). And what is revealed at that point can only be known by those who have been there.

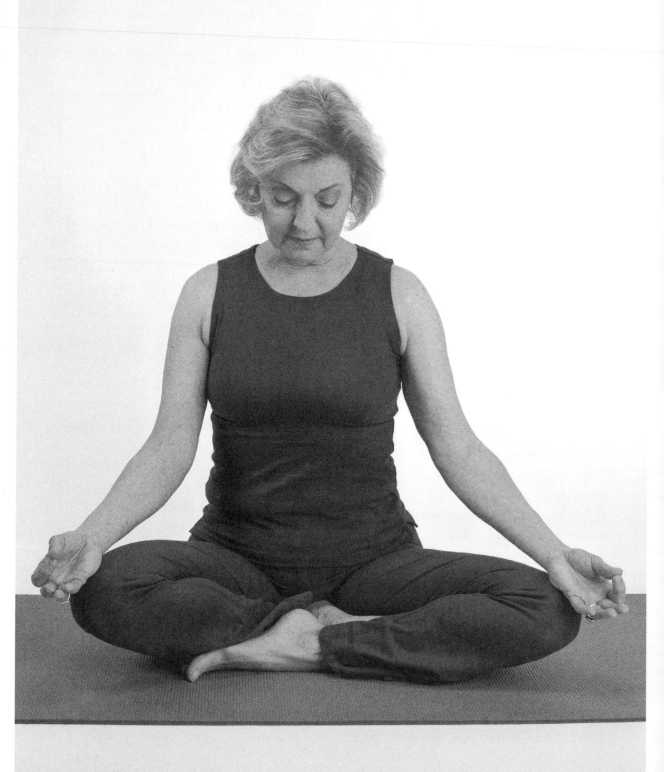

Chapter 8 AWARE PRESENCE

Hanging out in the Now with Meditation

I took my first-ever yoga *asana* class in 1971, back when I was living in Los Angeles and working as a biofeedback researcher. *Coincidentally,* (yeah, right!) the research center where I was working began the study of meditation. The projects we developed involved inviting people who claimed to be experienced meditators, coming from any number of spiritual traditions — Tibetan, yogic, Buddhist, Zen, and Christian contemplative — and connecting them to electroencephalographs (EEG), instruments that measure brain-wave activity, both frequency and amplitude, and then recording and observing the output, called brain "waves" of the neurons of the brain. What we came to notice as we worked with more and more people who had been meditating for years was that they all seemed be able to continuously focus their attention on one thing without distraction or interruption, as is the objective in meditation. If we introduced a noise or distraction into their environment (such as ringing a bell) their senses might notice it briefly but their attention wouldn't be pulled off their point of focus. On the other hand, in non-experienced meditators, any interruption would easily distract them and it would take a considerable length of time for them to get back on track.

We were able to notice these differences because the states of distraction or attention in the mind were actually measurable by the EEG instrumentation as a real-time printout of their brain-wave patterns. By "pattern" I mean a graphic interpretation of the mental activity that is recorded by the EEG as a result of very sensitive electrodes that are placed on a subject's head to pick up and *read* tiny electrical impulses of the brain. So we can *see* what has been going on in their head. This was very cool. Imagine a machine being able to tell you when you are distracted or focused!

As a result of uninterrupted focus, there were certain physiological changes that happened in the brain as well as in the rest of the nervous system and body. The brain-wave frequency began to slow down and the subjects seemed to "go" to very deep levels of consciousness, similar to the "unconscious" state of sleep, except they weren't asleep. They also showed a reduction in muscle tension, anxiety levels, heart rate, and respiration.

Let's see if we can look at what is actually going on here, especially with regard to the brain activity. When we are thinking, the thought process is a series of chemical reactions within the millions of neurons in the brain. I like to imagine that the brain cells function much like the process of internal combustion in an engine. Visualizing powerful, shiny, stainless steel cylinders in my car, going up and down at a furious pace, helps me to understand how the neurons of the brain might be operating! Each cell "fills up" with an electrochemical charge like the cylinders fill with fuel in the *intake* phase of combustion, then they "compress" and "fire" like the *compression* and *combustion* phase of the engine. And finally they "discharge," like the *exhaust* phase. Like buckets in a fire brigade, they fill and empty, fill and empty.

This process is thought itself, and it operates at a particular frequency. When you are thinking, or processing information, for example, like planning your vacation or recalling an unpleasant experience from earlier in the day, your brain neurons are actually operating at a frequency of somewhere between thirteen and thirty cycles per second. This is called "beta wave" activity and means that the neurons actually "fill" and "empty" between thirteen and thirty times per second. This is what is referred to as the "frequency" of the brain activity. The frequency, as well as the amplitude, of brain-wave movement is controlled by the autonomic nervous system, or what we used to call the "involuntary" nervous system.

Using a variety of parameters, we found that when we gave average subjects (not meditators) feedback or real-time information on what was going on in their bodies that normally their conscious mind wasn't privy to, most could learn some measure of control over this "involuntary" nervous system and manage to reduce muscle tension, alter their skin temperature, and change their emotional response to anxiety producing stimulus.

If we gave the subjects audio EEG feedback, for example, on a slightly slower frequency of brain-wave activity (equivalent to a light-level meditation) and asked them to try and increase the amount of feedback they were hearing, with practice most of them were able to increase the feedback, which meant they were slowing their minds down a bit and moving toward light meditation. Without the feedback, it was difficult for an average subject to have any idea of how to move towards the state of meditation without years and years of some kind of meditation training.

When we compared the charts of our ordinary subjects, being given the biofeedback training, with the charts of all the experienced meditators we had monitored, what we observed was that what the non-meditators were learning to do with feedback, the experienced yogis and Zen masters and monks seemed to be able to do *without* the biofeedback training. In states of authentic meditation, or "deeper" levels of consciousness, defined by the frequency of the brain-wave patterns — slower than thinking and similar to dream and deep sleep — heart rate and respiration slowed, muscles relaxed, blood flow to the hands and feet increased, and the frequency of the brain waves slowed down!

Our brain waves slow down when the thought

process slows down or ceases, as when we fall asleep. We could say that thought processes slow down when the frequency of our brain waves slows down. When we are awake, but relaxed and not thinking especially, the brain waves are slower than when we are thinking frantically. This is logical. Even if we never meditated or practiced biofeedback, we can sort of feel this slow down or shift in the speed of our mental activity. The totally amazing thing to me at that time, when we had these yogis hooked up to all this instrumentation, was that they could do all this slowing-down business without biofeedback training. They were able to slow their brain waves down to the place where most people fall asleep, yet they didn't fall asleep. How did they do this? Obviously, they had some kind of training, but what? This was totally new information for the medical world, but not so surprising to the yogis.

Under normal circumstances, your conscious mind isn't generally included when reports of the level of constriction or dilation in your peripheral arterial system, for example, are being passed around your nervous system. Why not? We couldn't possibly hold awareness of every single process that is going on in our body at this moment — like digestion, circulation, elimination, respiration, etc. So the body takes some of these processes and buries them a bit deeper under the control of the autonomic nervous system. But by bringing that information, via biofeedback, to the conscious mind, the brain can learn some level of control over that function. But what

does it take to make room for this awareness in our conscious mind? That is the key question, I think. It takes 1) making room in our mind for the information so we can absorb it without going into overload, and 2) turning off, or quieting the noisy cacophony of our mind so we can hear the subtle voice of the internal world.

UNDERSTANDING MEDITATION

Every form of meditation that I have studied since that time in late 1971 begins the training with some mention of, or focus on, the breath. Everyone who is alive breathes. It is a universally common denominator and familiar to all of us no matter what language we speak and no matter what religion we follow. Now, what is the reason that almost all forms of meditation begin with awareness of the breath? It is present. It's here. It's always in the present tense and if we train ourselves to pay attention to our breathing, it connects our mind to our body — the first step in integrating the subtle energy of soul with the gross matter of form. Now we are getting at it. But why do we want to meditate? Why do we have this desire to dig deeper into ourselves? And how does meditation help us to dig deeper exactly and see ourselves more clearly? Isn't just doing a little stretching and breathing enough?

Let's say as we are sitting quietly and starting to pay attention to our breathing, as we will do shortly, the first thing we begin to notice is our gross physical habits — like restless-ness. Is it physical discomfort that causes us to fidget and be uncomfortable with stillness or is it mental activity and stress? If we were to try and focus on our breath for five min-utes, what thoughts would intrude? Who or what takes our attention. This goes back to what we have discussed earlier in the previous chapter — what are you giving your energy to? What is taking your *prana*? If we started to do this five minutes every day, we would begin to notice this same restlessness in other areas of our lives. We would begin to look at all this stuff. What is going on with us — not only on the outside, but more importantly, on the inside? Where is our attention? Why can't we, for example, shut off our mind when we want to go to sleep? Under normal cir-cumstances, during the day we might not be aware of how busy our mind is, but when we want to sleep or meditate and the mind can't or won't shut off, suddenly we become aware of this restlessness.

Or perhaps we are terrible listeners. We don't know that we can't or don't listen until a friend or a partner tells us that we never lis-ten to them. Even then, we don't really hear this because we are busy thinking about our response and defense. As we continue this practice of trying to focus on our breathing for five minutes every day we start to notice more and more how our thoughts interrupt and how we are constantly distracted by mental fluctuations. This objective awareness of our restless mind is the first step towards beginning the practice of meditation. The

initial awareness that we are not our thoughts — in other words, what we are thinking about is not who we are, and that our thoughts are actually something that we can stand back from and observe — is the very first glimmer of awakening in the meditation process. The mental restlessness we experience is often called "monkey mind" in the yoga tradition, a phrase that graphically depicts an image of a monkey swinging around in the jungle from branch to branch, chasing whatever catches its attention. Literally, it refers to the mind jumping around like a monkey.

These fluctuations of our mind are caused by the going back and forth between the mental lists of what we desire and what we do not desire, or between what brings us pleasure (what is comfortable, enjoyable, and is to be pursued) and what we have an aversion to (what leads to unhappiness or discomfort and is to be avoided at any cost). Thinking about our desires and aversions creates a state of almost constant restlessness.

We spend a huge amount of time thinking about how we can maximize pleasure and minimize discomfort. Think for a minute about what you think about. No kidding. What did you spend most of today think-ing about? We are incredibly busy in this pursuit. We are going backwards in time, thinking about enjoyable things, and how to recreate them in the future. Or we are going backwards in time remembering unpleasant, painful events and putting our energy into manipulating the present so we can avoid having them happen again in the future. Now, this isn't all bad. It is a basic survival instinct — avoid things that cause pain, especially if they can kill you. But it is important that we practice *viveka* (discernment) and learn to distinguish between actual threats and mental distortions that we interpret as threats — which really are merely insults to our ego. Perhaps we have been criticized or misunderstood or disrespected — this is a normal part of life. It's gonna happen. We can't insulate ourselves from stress, from the 50 percent of life that is never going to be comfortable for us. All we can do is become comfortable with the uncomfortable — unless it's going to kill us. If it merely threatens our equipoise, we can move away, turn inward, focus on something else, or develop disregard.

With all this mental activity taking us into the past and the future there is little of us left over to actually experience life, as it is, in this moment. So how is meditation going to help with this? A meditation technique is designed to help us *learn to concentrate* on one thing, whether it is the breath, or a candle, or a sound, or an image. We are trying to learn to train the mind to focus on one thing and stay focused on that one thing. We cannot learn to meditate until we *learn to concentrate*. That is why *dharana* (concentration) is the sixth limb of classical yoga, and the first step of the *antaranga*, or the "inner limbs" of the yoga path, and *dhyana* (meditation) is the seventh limb. As we practice staying focused on one thing, we slowly get better at doing it, and as we learn to concentrate on one thing, the bodily processes, including thought, begin to

slow down. Every meditation technique has this one aspect in common: focus the mind on one thing, whether it is a narrow focus like repeating a *mantra* (a Sanskrit sound or word like *Om*, also written *Aum*) or an open focus like listening to *what is* (the sounds in the room, the rain, the bird calls, the thunder). The objective is the same — learn to concentrate. Look back at all the religious traditions and their scriptures, whether the Vedas, or the Koran, or the Bible. One thing they all have in common — every single authentic scripture tells us the same thing — and that is *to get your attention in present time*.

Why is this? Because it is only when we are present, in the moment, that we truly experience Life and can understand the wisdom of Universal Consciousness, or what in some religious traditions is called "knowing God." *Now* is all there is. *Now* is when we experience ourselves. *Now* is when we are happy. *Now* is also when we are unhappy. But both are simply opposite aspects of reality. And in the Non-dual, Universal Oneness, they are both just different sides of One Coin. We train the mind to pay attention through the practice of concentration so we can experience life as it truly is — as we manifest, experience, and express ourselves. As the mind learns to pay attention it becomes quiet. It is through this practice of stilling the mind that we begin to go deeper and deeper into ourselves and begin to realize our True Nature. *The understanding of the purpose and joy of meditation comes only out of the *practice* of meditation.*

Remember, the *experience* of meditation is

the *experience* of yoga, of finding that stillness within each of us that comes as a result of training the mind to focus. Meditation is not simply the repetition of the word or the counting of the breath—this is only preparation for the actual experience of meditation, as in *pranayama* or *dharana* practices. The meditation experience is the *full experiential reality of the present moment* that comes as result of the journey taken via the meditation technique. The technique is simply the boat that takes you across the river to the shores of the meditation experience itself. And just as when the surface of a lake becomes still like glass and you can see deeply into the depths of the lake, so it is when we go deeply into the stillness of the Self. The mind quiets and we find our connection to our soul or our True Self.

THREE MEDITATION TECHNIQUES

I have selected three different types of meditation techniques that we can choose among to move from our *pranayama* practice to the beginning work of developing a meditation practice. In one way, they broadly represent three quite different approaches to quieting the mind, but in another way, they are nearly identical in that they are taking us to the same place. Read all this over, and pick one that appeals to you. It is impossible to try and *lead* you through a meditation practice while you are *reading*! Obviously, you can't read this and actually *do* meditation at the same time. But what I have done is to write out what I would say in a guided verbal meditation if you were sitting in a workshop of mine. It's a little tricky. I would suggest that you read this all through once, just for an overview of how you settle in and make the mental transition from the outer world to the inner world. After having skimmed over the three various techniques, all of which begin and end in a similar way, you will have a rough idea of three different types of meditation and you might be in a better place to actually pick one technique to work with for yourself.

CONSCIOUS BREATHING

The first meditation technique we will work with in this chapter is Conscious Breathing. This is a simple and powerful technique that can be used by almost anyone at any time to relax, recharge, or reconnect with the present moment. It begins where our practice of *ujjayi pranayama* leaves off. But rather than using a specific breathing technique as we did in chapter 7 with *ujjayi* breathing, Conscious Breathing is simply the observation of our natural breath. In this *dharana* (concentration) exercise, we learn to recognize and make friends with the incessant chatter of the mind that we call "thought," which we have already been starting to do all through our *asana* and *pranayama* practices. The basic technique of this method was taught to me in California in the early '70s by Chogyam Trungpa Rinpoche. Over the years I have learned variations of this method from Thich Nhat Hahn, Pema Chodren, Charlotte Joko

Beck, and Alan Watts, and all these wonderful teachers have influenced my own teaching of this simple technique.

Conscious Breathing is the process of just sitting comfortably and allowing the attention to rest on the out-breath, like a bird rests on the branch of a tree after flying. It is a glorious way to relax — kind of like sliding into a warm, enveloping bath. The technique directs us to get our attention in present time, by turning our focus to our breath. This, in turn, leads us to notice more quickly, when we are "not" in the present moment, but rather are mentally drifting off to some distant time and place. It is this process of getting carried "off," that causes so much of our stress and anxiety and leads to stress-related illness and suffering. To recapture the essence of this moment, is to live our lives fully, spending our days with what "is" rather than frittering away our precious energy worrying about what "might be" or what has long since passed us by.

Conscious Breathing is an easy way to get grounded and centered. It affords us the opportunity to slow down and get in touch with just exactly what *is*, whatever that might be at the moment. As in *pranayama*, this technique further helps us to notice just exactly what we are doing with our *prana* or life force. As we sit, we start to realize that we can watch our thoughts, as something apart from our "self," as we might watch a movie. We begin to notice when exactly it is that we are distracted from the object of our meditation, which in this case is the breath. When we see a thought bubble up from the depths and pop up on the screen of our mind, we learn to recognize the thought as just "thought." Not good or bad thought, but just thought. We discover that we can pull our attention back from the past or the future and, delightfully, return to our breath and the present moment.

This is an uncomplicated practice that prepares us for more advanced meditation techniques. However, it is not a practice only for beginners. Even those of us who have practiced meditation for thirty or forty years can benefit from this technique, simply because this kind of work is so important and so easy.

REPETITION OF *MANTRA*

The second meditation technique is a form of meditation called *japa* or "recitation" in yoga. It refers to the repetition of a holy *mantra* (or sacred prayer) as the focus point for the mind. *Japa* yoga is a very old practice and is used by all of the great religions of the world. According to Georg Feuerstein, the American yoga scholar, this practice more than likely evolved out of the meditative recitation of the sacred texts by the priests and religious leaders in ancient times. It required great concentration by the monk or priest conducting the ceremony because every word had to be accurately pronounced so as not to adversely affect the sacramental ritual. Thus, it became a tool for developing concentration (or what we call *dharana* in yoga) and was passed along to the laity as a stepping stone to *dhyana*, or meditation.

Some *mantras* are only a few words, like the popular Roman Catholic prayer "Hail Mary, Full of Grace" or the Tibetan Buddhist Sanskrit *mantra*, "Om Mani Padme Hum." Others might be longer, like the Sanskrit *Gaiytri mantra*, which is several sentences long. No matter what the "prayer" or *mantra* might be, the objective in this type of meditation is to repeat the phrase or grouping of words over and over again either verbally or mentally. Often the practitioner will begin by chanting the *mantra* out loud for a time, in order to establish a rhythm of sound for the mind to follow, and then entrain the sound internally. Other times, the *mantra* is not "voiced" but is simply repeated over and over again mentally, going round and round like a tape loop.

For our *japa* meditation, I have chosen the simple mantra Om, one of the oldest and most sacred of all the *mantras* in Hinduism, Buddhism, and Jainism alike. According to *The Yoga Sutra*, the definitive text on the eight-limbed path of yoga, the word expressive of God, is *prananva*, or the symbol of Om. The Hindu Vedas say that the name of Brahman, or Absolute Divine Energy, is Om and Om is Brahman itself. Om is the primordial sound, the cosmic vibration. It is often alluded to as *pranava*, which literally means "humming." Om is the fundamental sound of the Universe and is present in every aspect, every dimension of the cosmos. *The Yoga Sutra* also recommends the recitation of the sacred syllable Om for the removal of all obstacles on the spiritual path. This practice, the *Sutra* tells us, will lead naturally to the contemplation and understanding of the inner significance of this *mantra*. It is not enough to simply sit and say Om over and over again like a parrot. Mindless repetition of *mantra* has no desirable affect. *Japa* must be performed with great attentiveness and reflection on its meaning.

SENDING AND RECEIVING

The third meditation technique is a classic and absolutely wonderful Tibetan Buddhist technique called *tonglen*, which means "sending and receiving." The groundwork for this meditation technique actually comes from the first practice of Conscious Breathing and is a meditation technique I have used for many, many years in moments of fear, loneliness, anxiety, or discomfort. This is an extraordinary technique that involves breathing "in" pain, or discomfort, and breathing "out" pleasure and relief. The idea can sound a bit daunting and depressing, but it is actually an incredibly uplifting and empowering technique. It immediately works to expand our normally narrow and self-centered outlook and helps to take us beyond the limited scope of our own ego. This is the longest and most challenging of the three techniques given here, but also one of the most beautiful and fulfilling. As with the two other techniques preceding it, and like most meditation techniques, this practice is what is called *adaptogenic*. In other words it is capable of raising or lowering the energy levels, depending on what is required at any given moment. It can pick us up if we are too lethargic or our energy is too *tamasic* (inactive), or chill us out if we are too frenetic or *rajasic* (active). Thus, these techniques can be used in time of feast or famine, drought or flood, scarcity or abundance, wellness or illness.

PREPARING FOR MEDITATION

To prepare for any of these three meditation techniques, it is important to select an environment with the least potential for distraction, just as we did for our *pranayama practice*. To review what we did in chapter 7 before beginning *pranayama,* this might mean that you close the door to your sitting room or meditation room or turn off the phone before you begin. It is also important to be warm and comfortable, but this doesn't mean curled up on the couch under a blanket. Perhaps, to stay warm, we place a cotton blanket or throw around our shoulders. We don't want to fall asleep. We look to sit up straight, with the chest lifted and the back held straight. This keeps the heart center open and receptive and the spine unimpeded for the movement of energy. We hold a position of alertness, but at the same time we want to be relaxed. If we are in pain, we will not be able to keep our attention on the object of our meditation practice — whether it is the breath, a mantra, or any other point of focus. Just as in our *asana* practice we look to find a place of poise between *sthira* and *sukha*, steadiness and comfort, hard and soft, so in meditation practice it is important to find the balance between tension and ease.

You may sit on a cushion on the floor or on a straight-backed chair, but either way, make sure that the seat is flat and not tilting forward or backward or to one side. If you are sitting in a chair, make sure that your feet are flat on the floor. If you are sitting on the floor, sit with your legs crossed comfortably in front of you in Easy Posture (or in lotus position or any other sitting posture that is comfortable). Sit quietly with the spine erect. If you are in a chair, do not lean back. If you are sitting on the floor, it is best to have your hips slightly higher than your knees. This might require placing an additional pillow under your buttocks to be more comfortable.

Close your eyes. Notice any little physical discomfort zones that might be taking your attention. Try to adjust them or work them out. Then reset yourself and get comfortable again. Rest your hands, palms face up, on your knees with your thumb and forefinger touching, or one upon the other in your lap, with the thumbs just touching. Relax your jaw, so that the mouth is almost open, with the tongue resting just behind the back of the upper teeth. Notice any restlessness. Take a few minutes to settle in.

Meditation is designed to quiet the mind and reveal the depth of human potential that resides in the heart of the soul. It is my wish that these techniques will come to be faithful old friends as they have been for me. It is important to eventually pick a meditation technique that you like, and that resonates with your spirit, and to then stick with it. Jumping from technique to technique will not take you to the depth of possibility that the practice of meditation is designed to create.

THE FIRST PRACTICE: CONSCIOUS BREATHING

Come to a comfortable seated position. Begin to settle. Take a few deep breaths. Notice any physical discomfort that might be taking your attention — any little crumb or pinch or tweak that calls out to you. Then make any adjustments in your posture necessary to come to physical tranquility. Work out any remaining kinks. Then settle again.

Now begin to notice the surrounding environment. What is going on today? Are the birds singing? Is someone showering? Noise? Traffic? Wind? Neighbors? Listen objectively. Try not to judge the sounds as good sounds or bad sounds. Just listen. Let them be. Accept them as part of what is for this moment. Notice the smell of the room. The feel of the air on your skin. Is the air cooler than your skin or warmer? Sit with this.

Now see if you can pull your attention "in" slightly and listen to the inner environment. What is going on there? What thoughts are taking your attention? Are you bored? Restless? Depressed? Excited? Irritated? Rerunning an event from earlier in the day? Who or what is taking your attention? Don't try to suppress or judge your thoughts. Let them bubble up from the floor of the unconscious mind. Watch your thoughts as if they were leaves floating by on the surface of a river. As you sit on the banks of the river, watch them as they pass by — in and out of view.

Now gently shift your attention to your breath. Ah, your breath. Are you able to just watch the breath without changing it in any way? This is almost impossible to do. Noticing the breath makes it conscious and inevitably changes it in some way. What is going on with the breath today? Take a moment to actually observe. Is it high or low? Deep or shallow? Rapid or slow? Labored or effortless? Stressed or relaxed? Have you ever watched a cat watch a bird or a dog watch a squirrel? Watch your breath like that now for a few moments as if it were the most interesting thing that you had ever seen.

Now begin to rest the attention on the out-breath. Just like that. Let the attention descend on the out-breath like the dry leaves flutter to the ground in autumn. Let the attention settle on the breath like a blanket of leaves. Gently falling and covering the breath. Inhale, relax and exhale . . . Just let your attention touch down for a moment and then go . . . Touch down and go . . . Feel the air on your skin. When you breathe in, it's like a pause or a gap. It's a little break, almost like a rising up, like a balloon lifting into the air. Then the attention floats down again to cover the out-breath. Rising up . . . resting . . . floating down . . . resting.

Nothing to force . . . No pushing . . . No

struggle. You cannot force the attention onto the breath. You must simply allow it to rest there, like the air is simply there, touching you. Holding you in every moment. Let the attention be like the air — gentle and effortless . . . just relax, as if you were falling towards sleep, but you do not fall asleep . . . the mind is alert and happy to rest on the breath.

Where is your attention now? Perhaps a thought has distracted you? Maybe you have wandered off a bit, following the thought as a puppy follows a butterfly. Oh! You suddenly become aware that you are no longer resting on your out-breath. As you notice this, let yourself smile softly and say quietly in your mind, as if you were recognizing an old friend . . . "Thinking!" and let the thought pass by. We don't judge the thought. We don't get mad at our mind. And we don't try to suppress the thought. We simply acknowledge the thought. Ah yes, there is the mind again. My wonderful mind, doing what it does best . . . "Thinking!" But now I wish to rest from thinking. Rest on the breath. Let the attention touch down on the out-breath as a butterfly lands softly on a blossom and then let it go. And again touch. And again let go . . . Again and again. Inhale, pause, exhale, touch.

Where is your attention now? Thinking! Every time the mind drifts off and you lose contact with the out-breath and you catch yourself in thought, simply say to yourself in your mind's voice, "Thinking!" and again come back to the exhalation.

Inhale, float.

Exhale, settle.

Notice the sounds that come to you from your environment. What are you hearing now? Still, the outside world is present. Inhale, pause. Exhale, settle. The air on your skin is so present, so complete. Thinking! Return. There is nothing to do except wait for the next out-breath. As that breath dissolves, we just wait, again, for the next moment, the next breath. Let the shoulders relax. Let the tension dissolve from the body. Exhale. Let the tightness give way to buoyancy. Exhale. Don't collapse your posture though, as you "sink" into relaxation and Conscious Breathing.

Slowly now begin your return journey to waking consciousness . . . Allow the gates to open, gradually bringing back in the outside world . . . Gently, quietly, the effortless effort to attend to the breath falls away. The attention begins to expand out, hearing, sensing, smelling. You're slowly returning to wakefulness. Begin gradually to move, twisting lightly first to the right and then to the left. Begin to open your eyes, halfway at first, letting the outside world return slowly. Then fully take in the light and the space around you. At a leisurely pace return to the world you left. Smile. Say thank you. Be grateful for this time and for all that you have. Carry this awareness with you for the rest of the day. Ommmmmmmmmm.

THE SECOND PRACTICE: CHANTING OM

Using *mantra* as a meditation technique is called *japa* yoga. This guided meditation will teach you how to use the sacred *mantra* Om as a point of focus for your meditation. However, before we begin to actually do this in the next program, we need to learn exactly how to use this *mantra* as a meditation tool. *Japa* yoga can be practiced verbally or mentally. Thus, we have the choice today of chanting the Om out loud or simply repeating it mentally in our mind. If we are going to chant the Om verbally, the sound is broken down into four parts — a, o, m, and *anahata*, or the sound that is beyond verbal pronunciation. Even if we wish to simply repeat the Om sound in our minds, it will be helpful to follow along here in order to learn the full expression of the *pranava*, or the universal sound of the Om. Learning the correct form for chanting *mantra* is a handy tool to have, whether in yoga class, in the shower, walking in the woods, or anytime by yourself.

A is the beginning. If you just hang your mouth open and make a sound, no matter what language you speak, it most likely will come out as an "ahhhhhhh" sound. This is the first part of the Om. The ahhhhhhh sound. Hear it in your breath. If you like, open your mouth and let the sound come out on the exhalation. Ahhhhhhh. The sound comes from the throat, way in the back of the mouth. Try it if you like. Just open your mouth and hum the "ahhhhhhh" sound. Try it again.

Ahhhhhhhhhhhhh.

In the second part, the sound moves forward to the hard palate at the roof of the mouth and the lips close to an "oh" position. Let's try it. Ahhhhhhhhooooooooooooooo. For the third part, the lips close and make the "m" sound. Feel the buzzing "mmmmm" vibration at your lips. Ahhhhhhhooooooooooooooooommmmmmmmmmmmmmmmmmmmmm. Now, for the last part, throw the hum up into the nasal cavity and the middle of the head, so it vibrates in your skull like the buzzing of a bee. Let the sound finish there. When the verbal sound ends, there is still a vibration, a buzzing sound that is always in you. This is called the *anahata*, or that which is "unstruck," or "unsounded." Practice this a few times. Try to give 25 percent of your total effort to each of the four portions of *prananva*, or the "humming" of Om. Now, let us move to the actual practice of *japa* yoga, or the repetition of the sacred *mantra* Om.

Whenever we chant Om, we are invoking Supreme Consciousness, or what some people call God. But Om isn't a specific God, only known to a few people in a particular religion. Om is generic, non-denominational, and without form or concept. In yoga philosophy, Om represents *Iśvara*, or the omniscient teacher's Teacher in yoga, the one who has known, who does know, and who will know everything. Om is the Supreme *Purusha*, the Lord of Yoga, the basic vibration of Universal Consciousness. Om is the seed sound from which all other sounds manifest. Sutras 26-28 in Book 1 of *The Yoga Sutra* state that "repetition of and reflection on the meaning of this symbol should be practiced, and its meaning will be revealed." This brings one-pointedness to the mind of the yogi. Om must be recited, as *The Yoga Sutra* tells us, with an appropriate meditative frame of mind. Then will follow the attainment of inward-mindedness and the disappearance of the obstacles.

Come to a comfortable, seated position. Sit with the spine straight and the chest lifted. Notice any little physical discomfort zones that might be taking your attention. Your knees? Your back? See if you can shift your posture to become more comfortable. Close your eyes. Rest your folded hands in your lap or on your knees. Then reset yourself and get comfortable again. Notice any restlessness. Take a few minutes to settle. Let any inner or outer physical distractions fall away.

At this very moment, there may be hundreds of thousands of beings around the world joining you in this meditation. Let yourself join this circle of Consciousness. The Om is the primordial sound, the fundamental reverberation of the Universe. It is present in every aspect, every particle, every nanosecond of Consciousness. In meditating on the Om, you are joining your Self to the cosmic vibration and to Absolute Divine Universal Energy. Sit with a noble heart and let your Self be worthy of this most auspicious time.

Bring your attention to the surrounding environment. What is going on? Take notice. Do you hear sounds? Rain falling? Wind blow-

ing? People talking? Accept the sounds as part of what is for this moment. Let them just be neutral. Not good sounds or bad sounds, but just sounds. Now bring your attention in and let it settle on the breath for a few moments . . . Inhaling and exhaling. Rising and falling.

Take a deep breath, fill the lungs completely, open the mouth and run through the four parts of the Om — from the "ah" at the back of the throat, to the "oh" in the middle of the mouth, to the "m" at the lips, and then to the hum in your head. Listen to the Om. Then inhale slowly, comfortably and sound out the a-o-m-mmm again. And again. Repeat this process over and over. If you are simply repeating the sound mentally, inhale and then, on your exhalation, let the Om sound begin. Coordinate your breathing with the mental sounding of Om. Let the sound go round and round.

Inhale, pause, Exhale Ommmmmmm. Inhale, pause, Exhale Ommmmmmm. Establish a rhythm, a beat, as if you were listening to music. Go round and round with the sounds, as if it were on a tape loop. Project the sound out into the world. Send it out to the other side of the room, then out the window to the end of the street, then on out to the edge of town. Keep projecting the sound, farther and farther out into the atmosphere. Break through the sound barrier and go on out into outer space. Pass planets and suns, meteorites and stars and galaxies. Let your sound dissolve into the sound of the Absolute.

THE THIRD PRACTICE: THE PRACTICE OF SENDING AND RECEIVING (*TONGLEN*)

The practice of *tonglen* is the practice of breathing in pain and breathing out relief. We begin this practice by focusing on something in our own lives that is painful. As we sit and attempt to quiet our minds and attend to our breathing, as we did in the practice of Conscious Breathing, perhaps some discomfort, some anxiety will take our attention. Perhaps it is something small, like a minor physical injury. Perhaps it is an embarrassment or a memory of something painful we endured. Perhaps it is something enormous, like the death of a loved one or the loss of our home through fire or hurricane. Instead of running away from the feeling of pain and hopelessness, and pretending it isn't there, which is what we normally do in life, we do the opposite. We allow our attention to settle on that very discomfort and try to breathe it "in."

Then we do an extraordinary thing. We breathe out comfort and relief. Again, we do the same thing. We breathe in tightness and limitation and breathe out spaciousness and freedom. As we breathe in the headache or the past insult or abuse or the loss, we imagine some kind of a transformational circuitry — maybe we flip upside down, or reverse direction or simply turn the discomfort over to the other side. Whichever way we choose to reverse the polarity of the in-breath, we do it. And then we breathe out relief.

Slowly, breath by breath, we inhale the fear, and then exhale the release of fear . . . Inhale contraction, exhale expansion . . . We breathe in the grasping and limitation. We breathe out letting go and limitlessness . . . Slowly, we begin to loosen our grip on our pain. Breathe in. Breathe out.

Now let us begin to *expand our circle of compassion* to include someone else suffering the same pain. We mentally reach out to someone else. Perhaps it is someone we know. Perhaps not. We breathe in their pain, their loss, their suffering. We breathe out relief and the subsiding of pain. Breathe in the pain, the loss for both of you . . . And breathe out relief . . . Breathe in loss . . . Breathe out fullness . . . Breathe in scarcity, breathe out abundance.

As we go deeper into the method, we keep expanding our circle of compassion until we take in all living beings everywhere. We breathe in suffering of all beings everywhere, experiencing the same pain. We breathe in the tragedy, breathe out light. We breathe in the claustrophobic fear, for example, of earthquake victims, of people alone and sick in hospitals, of the victims of war or abuse or anything you can think of, and then, as you feel your pain, their pain, all pain, breathe out liberation, space, and freedom from suffering.

We breathe in that which chokes us, scares us, paralyzes us, and breathe out spaciousness, connection, comfort, and movement. Slowly the grip of pain releases. We begin to loosen up a bit. Space enters. Time passes.

The healing begins. Our protective shield we have created to protect us from plunder and pillage begins to crack. We try to take refuge and hide from that which scares us but as we breathe, we find comfort in the protection of the unprotected state. Sit with this method for anywhere from twenty to forty minutes, depending on how much time you can take for this practice. Slowly bring your attention back to your natural breath. Sit for a few moments and decompress. This can be a very powerful meditation technique if you really get into it, so it is important to come out of your experience slowly and gently. You can set a quiet timer before you begin, so you know when your time for meditation practice is up.

If it would help you to follow a CD that guides you through all three of these three meditation techniques, please go to my Web sites, www.berylbenderbirch.com or www.boomer-yoga.com, to order *Everyday Mindfulness*.

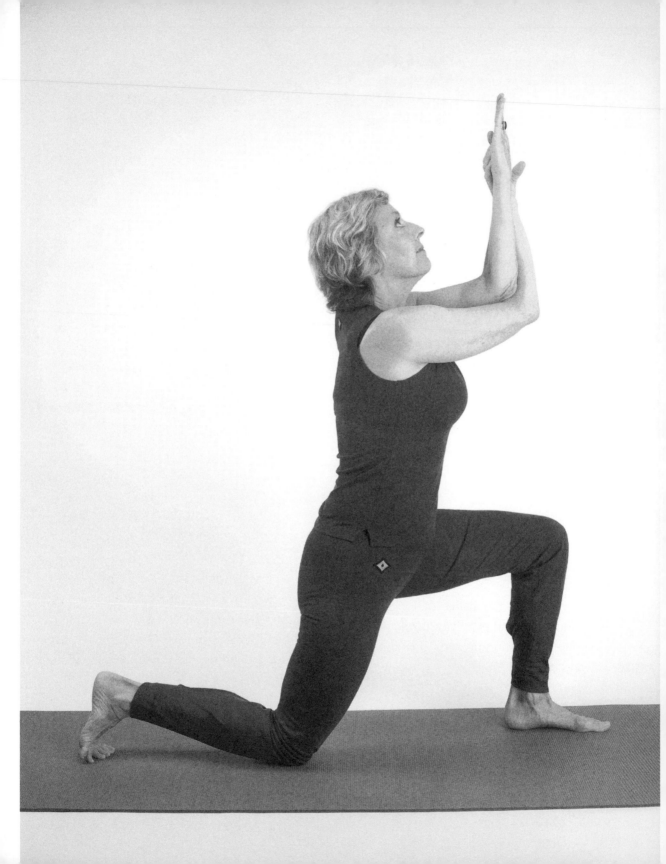

Chapter 9

SEEKING HIGHER SELF

The Journey Within

For most of our human history, the vast majority of human beings have taken it for granted that Nature is alive and that we live in a "living" world. That's a pretty important thing to acknowledge, and we are all descended from that very deep groove in our hard drive. Going back thousands of years — all the ancient cultures, the indigenous cultures — all of us collectively, regarded the entire cosmos as a vast living organism, just like a big animal, with a body and a soul. With some ups and downs and divergent streams of philosophical thought, this view continued from the early Greek civilization through to the earliest philosophy of Aristotle (384 BCE-322 BCE), and was passed along to subsequent generations — the heavy thinkers and scientists of the Middle Ages. The official doctrine in Europe of the Middle Ages was animism — the belief that Nature is alive, that the world is a living world — and had much in common with the animistic worldviews of all indigenous cultures. Can you remember that? If you space travel back through your previous lifetimes you should find that memory is imprinted in your DNA. But it sure has *gotten forgotten*!

Back in *those* days, if you were a scientist, you called yourself a "natural philosopher." Spirit and science were not separated. And even though you held a somewhat anthropocentric view of the world, believing that "man" and the Earth were at the center of the universe, you still had a sacred sort of regard for the world. Perhaps it was *because* you thought the Earth was at the center of things that, as a "natural philosopher," you were so spiritually connected to the Earth and the heavens and looked upon the cosmos as a living, breathing being, of which we were all a part.

For two thousand years, this way of thinking governed the way we as human beings thought about ourselves and our home, Planet Earth. Not only, though, did we think we were a part of this living, breathing organism, we thought we were smack dab in the middle of it. We got up in the morning and saw the sun rise. We went to bed at night and saw the sun set. Obviously, the sun revolved around us, the Earth, and so did all the other heavenly bodies in the Universe. Oh my. Talk about how our limited perception limits our ability to know Truth. But by the fifteenth and sixteenth centuries, the end of the Middle Ages, a shift was in the air. The way we humans looked at ourselves and our place in the cosmos was about to dramatically change.

What happened? Well, it was a hot and heavy time in science, and men like Copernicus, Galileo, Descartes, and Newton (remember them from your high school or college science classes?) made some pretty amazing discoveries over a period of about a hundred years — from late fifteenth century to the early seventeenth century — that sort of blew open our anthropocentric way of looking at things. They set down their theories and our view of our Universe and our home, sweet Planet Earth, changed from what it had been prior to the Middle Ages — we went from being *connected* to the living, breathing Earth and all life to feeling *disconnected* or separated from our Planet and one another, simply "cogs" in the Earth machine.

But how, exactly, did we get *disconnected*? Well, let's look at the big picture again. We have gone from regarding our world as *whole* and *alive* to seeing it as *separate* and *dead*. That's a huge paradigm shift. What happened back there in the late Middle Ages that changed our view of ourselves and our world so dramatically? It's a great story and it involves a little bit of history about those guys — Copernicus, Galilelo, and friends.

NOT THE CENTER OF THE UNIVERSE

Good ol' Copernicus, who we were taught in high school was the Father of Modern Astronomy, was really a bit of a bohemian. He was born in Poland in the late fifteenth century into a good Roman Catholic family. As a child he was fascinated by the stars and the heavens, and he would climb out his bedroom window and fall asleep on the roof watching the sky, until his mom came searching for him and tucked him back into bed. He became fascinated by astronomy when he first entered college in Krakow, and wanted to be an astronomer, but Dad wouldn't hear of it! His dad wanted him to go to Italy to study law and medicine, and then devote his life to the Church, so off he went to Rome to keep his dad happy.

Rome was a hotbed of intellectual life in those days, so as a young man in graduate school, Copernicus managed to do well enough to stay in school and still enjoy the electric and vital energy of southern Italy — a big change from Poland. Remember, this was the early 1500s! But he really didn't want to be a lawyer or a physician. One day, while hanging out in the equivalent of Starbucks of the day on the piazza in Doro (that's downtown Rome), through sheer synchronicity and good *karma*, he met the famous astronomer, Domenico Ferrara, and essentially, flipped out! This was his *dharma*! A real life astronomer! He became obsessed with Ferrara and squeezed time out of his studies to attend all Ferrara's lectures. He became an ardent disciple, spending hours gazing at the motions of the stars and planets with his *guru*, not dreaming idly as he had when he was a child, but making assiduous mathematical observations and documenting every inquiry.

By the early sixteenth century, Copernicus had figured out that that the Earth was not stationary, as had been assumed for thousands of years, and that it was not even the center of the Universe — it was just another planet going around the sun. He was smart enough to realize that this whole proposition of his seriously challenged the omnipotent authority of the Catholic Church and could get him into a truckload of trouble, not only with Dad, but with the Church. So he didn't say anything about his discoveries except to a few friends. For thirty years he kept his theories and ideas to himself.

But it wasn't just the overbearing theocracy of the times and fear of the Church's power that kept him quiet, but a subterranean angst that his work wasn't complete. He was always fiddling with his theories, I guess as any good scientist must do. He always felt his ideas needed reworking, which as it turns out, may have been a good thing for him because it delayed the release of his ideas. But one of *his* students kept bugging him to publish and he eventually completed and published his great work *De Revolutionibus* (you've read it, right?). The tome was a masterpiece and basically put forth a fantastic concept for the day — which was that the Earth rotated on its axis once daily and traveled around the sun once yearly! Isn't it hard to envision a time when people didn't know that? Imagine what we don't know today!

Well, this forever changed our view of the Universe and our place in it. We could no longer egocentrically think that we had greater importance than our fellow creatures, planets, and stars. We were simply part of the big picture, and (contrary to the Church theologians) not necessarily at the top of the heap.

GEOCENTRIC TO HELIOCENTRIC

I've always been a groupie for physicists and I'm sure in my previous lifetime somewhere I must have been sitting in a lecture hall, gaga over my hero, the Italian physicist, mathematician, and astronomer Galileo Galilei! He was the guy who invented the telescope in 1609 and, sitting night after night with his new invention, observing the heavens, he found evidence to support Copernicus's views. The position held by the Church was now on shaky ground, but so was Galileo, since he had observed that Venus circled the sun, and had discovered the orbiting "moons" of Jupiter. Throwing caution to the winds, he published his findings in 1610. Within two years, major opposition had surfaced in response to the theory of a sun-centered (heliocentric) solar system, which he supported.

The Church was furious with him and felt decidedly threatened. Consequently, as any powerful, fundamental religious authority would do, they judged his opinions to be dangerously close to sacrilege and forced him to retract his "heretical" heliocentric ideas.

Galileo apparently liked the idea of being alive. Aware that only a few years earlier the Italian philosopher, priest, and cosmologist Giordano Bruno, had been burned at the stake as a "heretic" by the Roman Inquisition for supporting Copernicus, Galileo very wisely decided to back down.

It was too bad about Bruno. He was a true mystic and deeply spiritual man. Although he supported Copernicus's work, he didn't feel any soul connection to Copernicus, but rather regarded him simply as a materialistic mathematician whose secular explanation and understanding of a sun-centered universe was just that — simply mathematical. He felt that his own understanding of heliocentrism was far more profound — perhaps it was. I would say that it is a safe bet to assume that Bruno's ideas were spiritually threatening to the Church and that's what got him burned at the stake. But either way, whether it was Bruno's mystical explanation or Copernicus's mathematical explanation of this Earth-going-around-the-sun business, the Church wasn't crazy about the idea.

I wonder if Bruno did yoga or practiced meditation. He must have had some kind of a strong spiritual, contemplative practice since, according to the history books, he believed in the Unity of all things and was strongly opposed to the Aristotelian notion of separating body and spirit. How did he figure that out? He encouraged humankind to achieve union with what he called "The Infinite One" in an infinite Universe. Sounds like the teachings of all the great Eastern Wisdom traditions, including yoga, as well as some of our modern mystics — like Mother Theresa and the Dalai Lama!

In his 2004 book, *Limitless Mind*, physicist Russell Targ reflects on the danger of offering scientific opinions contrary to the prevailing paradigm, whether today or four hundred years ago: "[It has] never exactly been a very popular stance with the ruling elite in any field, and even today it puts one in a similar position to the esteemed pioneers, Copernicus and Galileo (and Giordano Bruno), who suffered for offering correct, but *very unpopular* scientific opinions about the Earth's motion. To show that we were not special beings at the center of the Universe, as everyone believed, was not a view, to say the least, warmly welcomed by the Roman theocracy." Targ then goes on to quote Voltaire, "Commenting on this, Voltaire wrote, 'It is dangerous to be right in matters on which the established authorities are wrong!'" No kidding!!!

Boy, can I relate to that, having been thrown out of the "*ashtanga* church" after my book *Power Yoga* was published in 1995. I had been happily practicing a very traditional yoga method (the same I have been sharing with you in this book) for fifteen years and decided to "translate" the elite and esoteric methodology of the system into plain, simple, language that made it accessible for everyone — *ashtanga* yoga became "power" yoga. It was kind of like translating the Sacred Canon and Catholic Mass from Latin to Italian, so that the everyday man and woman on the street (who had always been told they had to go "through" the priests in order to talk to God, since God only spoke Latin) could now actually understand the scriptures and talk to God directly, without an intermediary! The Church didn't like that as it was too threatening to papal power, and neither did the primarily patriarchal "*ash-tan-ga*" theocracy when I wrote *Power Yoga*!

SIMPLICUS AND SALVIATI

Western Christian Biblical references say things like "the sun rises and sets and returns to its place (Ecclesiastes 1:5) and "the world is firmly established, it cannot be moved" (1 Chronicles 16:30). The seventeenth-century Church obviously took these scriptures very literally, not unlike the literal interpretation of some Biblical references by the Evangelical movement today. But Galileo didn't look at it that way and did not think his ideas were contrary to the scriptures. Like the different interpretations of the Bible that still exist today, he interpreted the scriptures in question more figuratively, like poetry and song, rather than as literal instruction and history.

He felt that the writers of the Bible were simply observing what they were able to "see," which was that the sun came up on one side of the Earth and went down on the other and therefore, they assumed it moved around the bottom of the Earth when it was out of sight. Although some interpretations of the Bible today regard the Bible as the explicit "word" of God, others conclude that it was not written by "God," but by a bunch of guys, not so unlike ourselves, sitting around a table drinking wine and trying to pass on the words of their guru, and decide what to include in the book. Not everyone agrees! Then or now.

In 1623 a good friend of Galileo's, Cardinal Barbineri, was elected Pope Urban VIII. He had been a longtime supporter of Galileo's work and he encouraged Galileo to publish again. The book Galileo eventually published ten years later was called *Dialogue Concerning the Two Chief World Systems* and in it presented his "new" theory, as well as the old traditionalist view of the universe. He wrote it as a theatrical debate between two characters — one of whom was mumbling and illogical and the other articulate and charming. Naturally, the first one presented the *traditional* view, and argued against Galileo and Copernicus. He was called Simplicius, and needless to say, appeared as an idiot. The other character, Salviati was cast in the part of the defender of the Copernicus and his sun-centered (heliocentric) viewpoint — to be played by a bright, good-looking Italian guy no doubt.

Galileo made the huge mistake of putting some of the words of his old friend, Barbineri, (who had become Pope Urban) into the character of Simplicus, the village idiot, and radically pissed off the Pope, who demanded a retraction and ordered Galileo to stand trial on suspicion of heresy in 1633. He was ordered imprisoned and later the sentence was commuted to house arrest, where he was to spend the remainder of his life. (You think things are tough now!)

FROM CONNECTED TO DISCONNECTED

Well, this set things rolling. The crack in the old paradigm was evident, and it wasn't long before it fell apart all together!! It seems that all through our cultural history, and continuing today, we have been propelled forward in our evolution when *who we think we are* begins to crumble and change — which of course it is always destined to do as long as *who we think we are* is based on something in the world of form. The very practical discovery that we weren't the center of the Universe, and the Church's reaction to anyone who agreed with that theory set the stage for the ideas of another guy we might remember from our high school physics class.

René Descartes, a philosopher, scientist, and writer, in the seventeenth century, became known for his famous quote, "I think therefore I am," (which we all know, as practicing yogis, is an illusion). He based his view of the world on a fundamental division between mind and matter and put them into two completely separate realms. This *Cartesian*

division was very handy for the scientists, who did not want — no way no how — to repeat the *errors* of Copernicus, Bruno, and Galileo and get themselves arrested or worse! The break-up of science and spirituality allowed them to treat matter as dead and completely separate from themselves, and to see the material world as a whole bunch of different parts pulled together into a huge machine. So they took up the position with gusto!! This kept the Church happy (*leave things of the mind to the Church*, was their thinking) and led to an extreme expression, in science as well as in culture, of the spirit/matter dichotomy.

The final blow to the old worldview was delivered by Sir Isaac Newton, physicist, mathematician, astronomer, and natural philosopher. He followed Descartes in his belief in the mechanical secularism of the world and was born the very same day that Galileo died. I sometimes wonder if he may not have been Galileo reincarnated, because he totally jumped on the same theories espoused by Galileo and Descartes, and once and for all cemented this dualistic view of the Universe. He regarded the world as a big, complex machine constructed of inanimate little parts that could easily be replaced if anything went wrong with the machine. He developed his famous Laws of Motion based on this separation between mind and matter. These laws became the foundation of classical physics and from the second half of the seventeenth century to the beginning of the twentieth century, the mechanistic, inanimate Newtonian model of the Universe and a rigorous determinism came to dominate all scientific thought. The entire cosmos, and particularly our planet, was no longer a living, breathing being, but rather, was reduced to a giant, inanimate machine.

God came to be viewed in science, and slowly in society as well, as an engineer who tinkered around with things when they needed to be fixed. The world was mechanized to the point where it denied life of any deeper meaning. Humans had no purpose and not much value. The view of a machinelike world, governed completely by universal mathematical laws, with no free will or spontaneity, was the essence of the mechanistic theory of Nature. As biologist and author Rupert Sheldrake has said, "This desacralized, deanimated, soulless vision of Nature became the foundation of modern science and was established as its reigning paradigm in the scientific revolution of the seventeenth century." Four European scientists and the discovery that we were not the center of the Universe, took us — in just a little over a century — from thousands of years of *connectedness to disconnectedness*! And we've been stuck with that for the past three hundred years.

But why, we might ask, did it go this way? Why did human evolution go through the mechanical period of Newtonian physics? What was the point? Was it a detour that led us into the unfortunate conditions of alienation and isolation? Well, for starters, it wasn't a mistake. If we hadn't gone through "old" physics, we couldn't have arrived at "new" physics, just as in yoga, *asana* leads to meditation. Nothing in this world happens "by mistake," and things never are just all good or all bad. This may seem a little obvious, but once something happens, it's part of history. Whether we view a situation as a "good" event or "bad" event, there is no doubt it had a place and a purpose. Plus, it is practically impossible for anything to happen that is all bad from all points of view. Given time and perspective, we come to see that there is some aspect to most events that helps to propel us forward, bringing change and, sooner or later, growth and greater awareness.

We can certainly begin to see a relationship between this new paradigm put in place by Newton's theories and the breakdown of a homogeneous culture, and the ultimate secular disregard for our Mother Earth. It makes sense to me that the entire mess we are in as a species and as a planet, can be traced to this mechanistic idea of thinking of the planet as a big machine, in which if anything broke down, ran out, or came unhinged, it could just be replaced with another part. Our TV or computer or cell phone is old or broken — no problem, throw it out and get a new one. Our disregard for the Earth, our willingness to pollute and use up our non-renewable resources, our lack of respect for our forests and wilderness, and most importantly, our insolence towards other species, indicates that we are missing an important respect for the Universe and its contents as part of *life* and part of the big picture.

A paradigm, which is simply a set of assumptions, a school of thought, starts to shift when, as physicist Peter Russell says in his 2002 book *From Science to God*, "Some brave soul (or souls) challenges the beliefs behind the existing worldview and proposes a new model of reality." For thousands of years, things we regarded as connected and inseparable now became simply parts of a machine that could be disconnected and replaced. This was a pretty big shift. How did this paradigm shift affect us as a society? Well, slowly we began to partition ourselves into fragments and came to see ourselves as separate and interchangeable parts of the whole. As this idea became rooted in our collective worldview and social structure, it initiated and perpetuated even more separation.

There are advantages to division — such as the ability to specialize and focus on specifics. Take a group of people and give them a problem to solve. Split them up and then ask them to focus on different aspects of the problem. The solution will be far more creative and broad than if they had all just looked at the overall dilemma. So as a society we have benefited from this specialization — particularly in the areas of technology and medicine. Think about cell phones and digital photography and MRI's and touch screens! The splitting up of science, for example, into various fields such as physics, chemistry, biology, neurobiology, zoology, etc., has made it possible for various groups of people to focus exclusively on one particular aspect of investigation, and we have all benefited from what is called this *reductionist* approach to advancing knowledge. But there are also massive disadvantages of fragmentation. As we can see by just looking around, it can eventually lead to alienation from the rest of the pack. We recognize, both in science and in our culture, entire segments that live out their whole lives in a shell, without any awareness of what is going on in other segments. As the great philosopher and Indian sage Krishnamurti says, "A problem only arises when life is seen fragmentarily, do see the beauty of that."

So here we are — arrived in the twenty-first century — separated, alienated, and isolated. You personally, reading this now, may not feel alienated or isolated, but as a culture I think, most people do. We have become replaceable cogs in the wheel. In medicine, we see the body regarded, not really as a whole system, in its totality, but as a collection of parts. You can confirm this notion for yourself if you have a medical problem that needs to be diagnosed. You will, firsthand, experience the reductionism in the world of medicine, when you find that your gynecologist doesn't talk to your gastroenterologist who doesn't talk to your orthopedist, who doesn't talk to your rheumatologist who doesn't talk to your neurologist. They will all repeat the same tests, unless you hook them up. The hooking up part is totally up to you. Everything is fragmented.

THE SEEDS OF VIOLENCE

We see on TV and hear on the radio about war and massacre and genocide taking place in different countries around the world. We look at it and shake our heads and wonder how in the world we got to such a mess. How can the politicians do this? What is wrong with *those people over there*? Why doesn't someone stop all this? Almost all of us have this reaction. I don't know too many people who jump up and down over the prospect of war, and those who do, at least in the Western world, generally are not sending there own biological sons and daughters off to fight! Indian spiritual master Vimala Thakar asks the question in her 1984 book *Spirituality and Social Action: A Holistic Approach*, "Where are the roots of war? Are they just in the minds of a handful of individuals ruling over their respective countries, like Korea, or China, or Iraq, or Afghanistan, or Russia, or even the U.S.? Or are the roots of war in the systems that we have created and have been living for centuries — the economic, the political, the administrative, the industrial systems? . . . If we go deep, won't we find the roots of war in the systems and structures that we have created?"

The truth is that violence begins with us. And it comes from our mistaken view of ourselves as separate. We have accepted violence — in our media, in our entertainment, in our children's games, in our relations with other countries and other religions, and in our way of living altogether. We have to accept responsibility for our complicity and for how we cooperate and participate in the systems and thereby participate in the wars and the violence. If we search and question ourselves and go to the roots of the problem we will see that we are expressions of the collective unconscious. The seeds of violence and the source of human conflict begin deep within us — in the human psyche. It's like a Möbius strip: our social structures and systems have conditioned our inner belief systems and perceptions and those inner beliefs and perceptions then further create and perpetuate the systems and structures. It is important for us to recognize that these two seemingly different worlds are intertwined and we cannot just try to fix one part — they are inseparable. So how do we break into this loop?

RETURN TO WHOLENESS

When we begin to practice yoga, we begin to develop a greater awareness of not only our inner beliefs and how they shape our behavior, but of our social structures as well. We break into this loop with *aware presence*. We start to see — little momentary glimpses of how violence begins with us, not those folks over there. But I don't think we can see that before we go through some of the early stages of our spiritual training. It is important to realize that there are certainly other paths besides yoga that can be taken for personal evolution and spiritual growth. Yoga isn't the only way but it is one way that is authentic, has lasted over the centuries, and is accessible today, providing an effective map to the awakened state.

We started with *asana*, and then *pranayama*, and that work began to clear the path to greater clear-seeing! Remember I said earlier that even though *ahimsa* (non-violence) was one of the five *yamas*, which, as the first limb of the eight-limbed path provides the fundamental groundwork for our practice, we generally need to do a little basic work with the more gross aspects of the practice before we can see how *ahimsa* or any of the other *yamas* play out in our life. As we begin to *practice* yoga, and work at being present with what *is*, it wakes us up and we become better able to see ourselves from a distance, to see what takes our attention, what we do, and how what we think, which previously was mostly unconscious. We become less unconscious, a little more aware of how we separate ourselves and label some pieces of our life's puzzle as good, and some as bad, some as friends, some as enemies, some as comfortable, and some as uncomfortable. Since we've got puzzle pieces all over the place, we begin to understand why we can't see the completed puzzle in its Oneness.

As we start to become more aware of how we are internally divided, and how we divvy up the world around us into endless parts, and we start to realize how untogether, uncomfortable, disconnected, and alone that makes us feel, we begin to do it less. With every conscious breath we take, as we've been learning to do with our practice, we begin to understand change and impermanence a little better, and that what appears to be fragmented is in *reality* connected. Everything is connected. How could it be otherwise? It is only our distinction between what we like and don't like that breaks things into pieces.

Recently I heard a program on National Public Radio talking about the recent dramatic growth, in this country anyway, of organic farms, community food cooperatives, and farmer's markets. People are going back to the source, to smaller, local producers to feel more connected to their food source. Apples, grown locally and picked yesterday, seem to have a stronger soul connection to our tummies than those sprayed, produced-for-maximum-shelf-life-in-Styrofoam-plastic-convenience-packaging, lifeless, tasteless looking things they *call* apples. There is a movement. Can't you feel it? What is going on?

A new worldview is emerging and another shift is happening *now*, from *disconnected* back to *connected*. Ironically, once again, the shift is being pushed along as a result of the new findings in science. But it's a little different from the position of six hundred to two thousand years ago, when the belief of the cosmos as a living, breathing, inseparable organism was based on intuition and just plain heart connection to the spiritual realms and prevalent worldview. Now, this connectedness is based on very sophisticated mathematical formalism, coming out of quantum theory, or the "new" physics. As I have heard the biologist Rupert Sheldrake say, "We are living through a major period of change in science, a paradigm shift, from the idea of nature as inanimate and mechanical to a new understanding of nature as organic and alive. The God of a living world is very different from the God of a world machine."

But the shift I think is also happening as a result of something else that is running concurrently with the revelations occurring in quantum physics. And you may already have begun to guess for yourself what that might be! As I have said many times in workshops, it is no mistake that the *science* of yoga is here now, and being embraced by people all over the world. The availability of the teachings and methodologies of the Eastern Wisdom traditions, one of which is yoga, are significantly contributing to the shift back to Oneness that we have been missing for so long — in our science, in our culture, and in our hearts.

Ever since Newtonian mechanics became the reigning scientific paradigm, science has held two basic assumptions about the world: 1) that there really is "something" out there — in other words, there really is a material world, and 2) that this "something" is non-living or insentient. As noted physicist Fritjof Capra writes in his book, *The Tao of Physics*, "Questions about the essential nature of things were answered in classical physics by the Newtonian model of the universe which reduced all phenomena to the interaction of hard, material, insentient, indestructible atoms." Even today, there is still a large group of conventional physicists holding to the old paradigm and trying to explain the unfolding of the universe in materialist terms. But more and more these answers don't fit.

And they don't fit primarily because of the troublesome concept of Consciousness. Hmmm, this definitely poses a problem. Newton, as we saw, just decided to sidestep the whole issue. Consciousness didn't seem to be composed of *matter,* and just didn't fit into the equations. So it was best to just leave it out — leave it to the philosophers and the Church. "We scientists will focus on matter and the material world." But as modern physics, with the aid of modern technology, has probed deeper and deeper into this essential subatomic world, the possibility of leaving Consciousness "out" doesn't work any more.

At the frontiers of science today, in research being done by people like Harvard-trained quantum physicist Michio Kaku, scientists are beginning to discover that the Universe itself is functioning as if it were a living system, and the idea of the cosmos as a lifeless machine has surrendered to the representation of the cosmos as a living, breathing, organism! Social scientist and evolutionary activist Duane Elgin, and author of the classic 1981 book, *Voluntary Simplicity*, has said when talking about several trends that herald new opportunities for our collective evolution — that "the physics theory of non-locality tells us that the universe is connected with itself, despite its enormous size. Also, Consciousness appears to be present at every level of the Universe, from the subatomic scale on up."

It's pretty exciting to think that a growing number of scientists, who are trying to explain Consciousness, are beginning to think like yogis and mystics. They are moving out of the old worldview and realizing that it is not possible to explain something that is intangible within a worldview that is intrinsically materialistic, or to fit many of the new findings into neat mathematical equations.

In many areas of science, but particularly in physics and cosmology, the idea of the *field* has replaced the old, pre-Newtonian role of the "soul." The idea that Nature is inanimate has been replaced by the theory that Nature, or *prakriti*, as it is called in yoga philosophy, is organized by *field*. Like souls, *fields* are invisible organizing principles. Our body is a *field*, as we talked about in chapter 2, not a solid, unchanging clump of matter, and it exists within a bigger *field* — the Universe.

The complete ongoing evolution of science, whether mechanically driven or not, is all an intentional, ordered part of a Great Holographic Design that is growing, changing, and very much alive. Even the contributions of Newton and Descartes, which are sometimes regarded with disdain by modern physicists for their emphasis on mechaniza-

tion, were not a mistake. Ironically, it is the competition, specialization, and this very mechanization in science and culture that has rocketed us to the new frontiers, and is leading us back to *connectedness*. In quantum theory, this idea of *connectedness* is called an emergent property. How odd. How can something be *emergent* that has always been? Maybe *emergent* is being used in the sense that most of us here in the relative world are unaware of it. That doesn't mean that it doesn't exist and hasn't always been in effect. On the contrary, it simply means that a small percentage of humankind is in the process of "discovering" it and the rest of society is still stuck in the old paradigm, and still sleeping.

By "sleeping" I mean "not awake" and stuck in the isolated and materialistic struggle for stuff and security. As Buddha says in Deepak Chopra's book *Buddha*, "The human predicament — everyone is asleep, totally unconscious about their true nature. Some catch scattered glimpses and go back to sleep. The bulk of human beings had no glimpse of reality. How can they know? *You are all Buddha.*"

CONNECTEDNESS EMERGING

We have worked our butts off to find some sense of physical security, economic security, comfort, entertainment, etc. And then we have to continue to work to protect and hang on to what we have! We think "we've got it and we're going to keep it." And we are certainly going to keep anyone else from "getting it." So we continue to face internal conflict, confusion, uncertainty, prejudice, jealousy, and fear. And as long as we continue, as humankind, to identify only with the world of change, and expect it to be permanent, we will constantly recreate suffering for ourselves and everyone else.

I think on some level we must intuitively know that none of these things we have, offer real security. Only when we know who we truly are, when we experience the True Self, can we find the security we seek. This True Self is discovered at the end of a spiritual journey — it does not reveal itself in the world of stuff, the world of change. Until then we have no ground to stand on, no firm foundation, and over and over, as what we think is permanent and will not change does change, we are left thrashing around in the deep water looking for a raft. If we can't get ourselves together then how can we see the wholeness of the world?

As we blow apart the obstacles and dig our way into the depths of the collective unconscious, with this incredibly methodology called yoga, we will see that there is nothing fundamental that differentiates any one of us from another or, really, from any sentient being! We are *connected* and more and more people are realizing it. That is Self-realization — the realization of the Self, of the One, of the No Boundaries! If Detroit pumps out excessive carbon dioxide into the atmosphere, it isn't just Detroit's problem. The CO^2 is disseminated in the atmosphere and it circles the Earth. It is our atmosphere, One Atmosphere, One Planet. It is our problem, One Problem. We are living the reductionist paradigm, but we cannot escape the fact that we are bonded together.

And how are we ever going to realize this, to realize our collective Self? Well, some groups are working from the angle of changing the external systems and structures, like, hopefully the Obama administration will do. Others, like many of us, are doing it through our work with this book, toiling to change the inner belief systems. It appears that we could go either way and both paths are important.

THE ARISING OF CONSCIOUSNESS

So here we are I think — today — at a point in our history, a moment, when what I have been pursuing my entire life — the omega point – the zenith where science and philosophy, physics and metaphysics come together — is emerging. It is so exciting. It's an incredibly brilliant time to be embodied and conscious! One time back in the early seventies I heard Swami Satchidananda, the founder of Integral Yoga, say, "Consciousness is the field of all possibility." At the time I thought that that meant that if you were "conscious" you could do anything. Then, many years later, I heard the physicist Peter Russell quote the *same words* from Satchidananda and it lit up the memory banks in my brain. But all of a sudden I *heard* it in a completely different way! Wow. Consciousness is the *field* of everything. Everything is a construct of Consciousness, the *Field* of all possibility, the Big Void. It was a completely new understanding of exactly the same words. Maybe thirty years had passed.

Once we break through the limitations of the perceptual boundaries of the sense organs, it is possible to realize the absolute boundless nature of the Universe. That penetration can occur in several different ways such as through a peak experience, like extreme grief or joy, or through a spiritual discipline like yoga, for instance. In fact, that is what the yoga path is all about, a tangible methodology for the quieting of the mind activity and the turning inward of the senses. Yoga is a means for going beyond the limitations of the senses, shining the light on the inner world. The resulting experience, when this quieting of the mind actually happens, is the actual *experience* of yoga. Realization of that state of connectedness, or boundlessness, can occur, as it did for me initially (and for many of the children of the '60s), through the aid of a psychedelic plant, or through meditation, or through just plain dumb luck (although in the big picture it isn't dumb luck — it's been planned for eons). But up until that point, we are in bondage to our senses and their limitations.

From the time we are born our senses feed us information, and the way we receive that information in our sense receptors and the way in which we are taught to interpret that data, determines what psychologists call *premature cognitive commitment*. In other words, we buy into the world of our senses and assign that perception as our reality.

As an infant, I see Mommy sitting "over there." There is "space" between us. That's what my eyes tell me. Mommy is wearing a "blue" dress. I am taught that the "color" I see — the light reflecting off Mommy's dress — is blue. I carry that mindset out into the world. We set ourselves at the center of our world. With very well-defined conceptual boundaries of both body and mind. Everything else is "out there." But the truth is that we are not separate and we are not in the center of our world. And there may well be "nothing" out there!

Everything is an arising of Consciousness. Try to fashion an image in your mind of what that might mean??? Everything is an arising of Consciousness? What that means is that every experience, every thought, every idea, every situation, every living being, every tree, every song, anything you can conceive or create — all of it — is all fashioned from an arising of Consciousness. Aldous Huxley has described this concept in his *perennial philosophy*, which was a term he used to describe the highest common factor present among all the major wisdom traditions and religions. The first principle of his philosophy was that Consciousness is the major building block of the Universe. He believed that our purpose in life is to become one with what he called, God, what we might call Great Spirit or One Taste, or Absolute Universal Consciousness. Isn't that what yoga is leading us to — the True Self? Who is the True Self if not God?

What makes us ultimately and finally happy? Answering the question, Who Am I? and discovering our True Self, which is none other than Aware Presence, or God (I like to say the Present Moment because *here* is the only place we can ever be and *now* is the only time we can experience God). Ahhhhhhhhhh. Knowing the Self opens the heart and awakens compassion and that feels good and brings lasting happiness. And yoga is trying to teach us that there is only One of us here — the individual consciousness (*Atman*) and the universal consciousness (*Brahman*) are One!! The famous physicist Erwin Schrodinger, who perfected quantum mechanics, thought that that teaching of yoga, equating *Atman* and *Brahman* to be the "grandest of thoughts."

This idea of everything coming up out of the primordial soup of Consciousness is impossible to conceptualize. So then how do you begin to understand it? The way I think of it is via metaphor. I imagine cooking chocolate pudding. Or, if you have never cooked pudding, visualize the viscous muddy hot springs at Yellowstone National Park. As the pudding thickens, and begins to heat up, little mounds of pudding rise up, pushed by bubbles of steam coming up through the mixture, and make little bursts through the surface. Poof, a spray of steam hisses into the air. Ahhh, Consciousness arising I think to myself. Everything in the Universe comes out of that pot of pudding, bursting forth.

If we are going to say that everything is made of Consciousness, well, what is Consciousness made of? So, we ask, what is the underlying, fundamental element of this basic building block that apparently makes up everything? Well, science has been trying to figure out the answer to that question for hundreds of years. Of course, the only way to really "study" Consciousness is to sit down, get still, and go *in* and take a look at what is going on inside. This is what the ancient seers and *rishis* and saints and spiritual adepts did in order to figure out the nature of the Universe and to come to the extraordinary realizations that they did about the non-local, indeterminate, linked nature of every part of the Universe with every other part. And it is what you have been doing with your work in the past eight chapters — focusing your attention, getting still, going in and taking a look around the inner world.

It has always been apparent to me that everything was sort of connected in one big swirling mass of something or other — emptiness, maybe, but not nothingness. Well, not always apparent, I guess. I think I was born feeling connected on some level. I felt it at a very early age, and then the feeling disappeared for about twenty-five years or so. When I was three or four I would sit on a rock in the woods with my imaginary totem animals, a wolf, a jaguar, and a dragon fly, all friends and constant companions, at my side, and be motionless for hours at a time, with my eyes closed, going "in" — time traveling, shape shifting. Going backwards and forwards in "time," but always being "here." It's a little tricky to describe, but I vaguely remember the feelings.

ONE MORE THING

"He threw the dust into the air; it remained suspended like a murky cloud for a second before the breeze carried it away. 'The dust holds its shape for a fleeting moment when I throw it into the air, as the body holds its shape for this brief lifetime. When the wind makes it disappear, where does the dust go? It returns to its source, the Earth. In the future that same dust allows grass to grow, and it enters a deer that eats the grass. The animal dies and turns to dust. Now imagine that the dust comes to you and asks, 'Who am I?' What will you tell it? Dust is alive in a plant but dead as it lies in the road under our feet. It moves in an animal but is still when buried in the depths of the Earth. Dust encompasses life and death at the same time. So if you answer the question 'Who am I?' with anything but a complete answer, you have made a mistake.'"

— Deepak Chopra, *Buddha*

I could fly at will — just lift off with a slight concentration of effort — and did frequently. Once I broke free of gravity, it was easy to gain altitude. I went to the edges of the Universe I am sure, moving through some invisible *field*, that we all were part of on some very fundamental level. But then, as I grew older and the reality of social construct closed in, I forgot who I truly was, and entered a state of *maya*, like most of us. I became trapped by my thoughts about who I was and by the boundaries and artifacts of sensory perception. The world was this material place and I was a thing in the world. I became my body. I became a daughter, a student, a singer in the choir, a pretty baton twirler, a good cheerleader, a bad actor, a success, a failure, a photographer, a waitress, a Playboy bunny, and on it went. Who I was, was whatever it was I was thinking about at any given moment, or whatever descriptive term I happened to assign myself at the time.

WHO AM I?

But as I evolved a bit through an almost forty-year practice, grew older and a bit wiser, and became more aware, I came to realize that who we are is *not* what we are thinking about, or what we have, or what we know, or who we know, etc. So we ask the really big question, *Who Am I?* And there is only one place to answer this question, and that is in the stillness of your own mind. How do we get to that place? Only one way, we work to get our attention in present time — exclusively. That quiets the surface noise of the internal world and let's us go down to the depths, where the answer to *Who Am I?* resides. How do we find higher Self? I can't really tell you or even take you there, but I can say that the journey you have been following through your life and through this book, hopefully, will set you on an authentic quest for the answer, and hopefully to an *experience* of the answer. It isn't the only way, by any means. It may not even be the best or fastest way. But it is an authentic path. It is the methodology of classical yoga. Just practice and the rest will fall in place. And you will only know what I am talking about once you get on the train and get going!

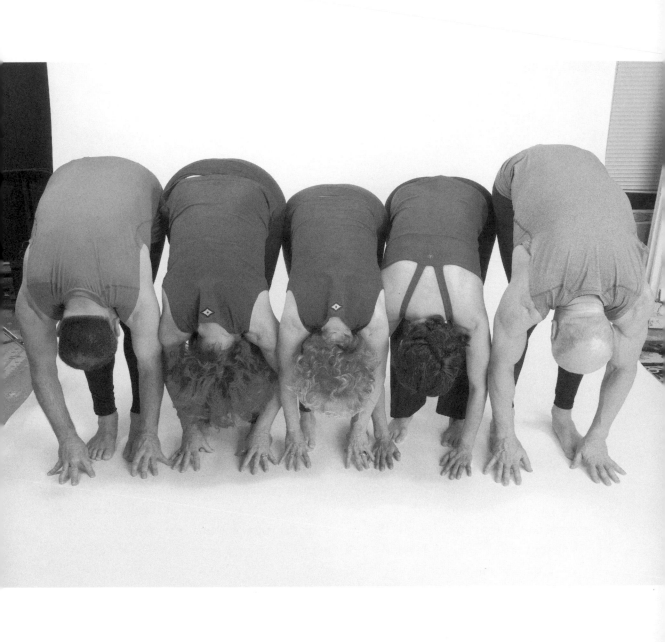

Chapter 10 GIVING BACK

On Becoming a Spiritual Revolutionary

What is our work in the world? What is our ultimate purpose? The Dalai Lama answered, when asked this question, "To be happy." I was surprised. I thought he would have said something like, "To help reduce suffering and violence in the world." But, no, he said our ultimate purpose was to be happy. Every living thing wants to be content, and well, yes, *happy*. What makes us happy? Well, deep in *The Yoga Sutra*, Patanjali gives us the answers we are seeking and delineates "the work" we need to do to find lasting happiness.

In Book 1 of *The Yoga Sutra*, the most esoteric of the four chapters, Patanjali "defines" yoga as "the cessation of the fluctuations of the mind." This isn't really a definition, but more a road sign that says, "Go this way. Quiet the mind and you will experience yoga." Yoga isn't the quieting of the mind; it's what happens when the mind is quiet! If we want to have the *experience* of yoga, we need to still the fluctuations (or the thoughts) of the mind. So how do we do that?

Okay, so Patanjali goes on to say that these modifications (or thoughts — *vrittis* in Sanskrit) of the mind can be controlled by two things — *abhyasa* (practice) and *vairagya*

(non-attachment). And if we can get these two things in place they will take us to the experience of yoga. Okay, well, that's a help. I think at this point you have a pretty good idea of what, in yoga, is meant by *practice*. What about *non-attachment*? That doesn't sound too inviting. Actually, non-attachment is simply the release of craving. It doesn't mean passivity or non-involvement in life. It means not clinging, because as yogis we know that everything in the world of form will eventually pass away — so we appreciate things and life as they are, in this moment, and learn not to hang onto them for dear life. Ha. That sounds like a good trick. How exactly do we develop *non-attachment* and *practice*?

Well, in the very first sutra of Book 2, the most practical of the four chapters, Patanjali tells us. He defines what is called *kriya yoga*, or the yoga of action, the yoga of work. This pro-active yoga method called *kriya*, is comprised of the last three of the five *niyamas* that I began to identify in chapter 7 — *tapas*, *svadhaya*, and *Iśvara pranidhana*. Here he gives us the secret to developing *practice* and non-attachment! How do we find happiness? We do the work of yoga!!!

First, we need to clean out the sludge. *Tapas* literally means "heat, or to burn; austerity." The practice of *asana* is considered a means for burning off toxins and impurities and is an expression of *tapas*. We've got that one already going on. What's next? Second, we need to study. *Svadhaya* means "study" in the context of the spiritual teachings, which is what you are doing through the reading of this book. And the third aspect of *kriya yoga* is *Iśvara pranidhana*. *Pranidhana* means "surrender" to *Iśvara*. *Iśvara* is the Supreme *Purusha*. *Purusha* is the opposite of *prakriti*, which as you may remember, means the world of form or Nature. So what is *Purusha*? Great Spirit, God, Aware Presence, Absolute Consciousness. How do we surrender to something so non-conceptual? Well, to me, as I said earlier in the book, it means surrender to the Present Moment. Get your attention in present time. What is the work then? What is the secret yoga code to happiness? Do the work — sweat, study, and surrender to this moment. That's it.

CELEBRATE IMPERMANENCE

A powerful part of the week-long yoga teacher trainings that my school directs is a ritual called Celebrate Impermanence. The group of students, early in the week, creates a "Council of Elders," which is simply a way of bonding with other participants, committing to the work, and agreeing to be a participatory and equal member of the "council." In addition to early morning *asana*, *pranayama*, and meditation, a good part of our training is spent in study of *The Yoga Sutra*, and a good part of that is dissecting the meanings of *practice* and good ol' *non-attachment*! I ask everyone in the group to name something that they are attached to. Then we acknowledge that everything we have named, from family to work to health, we will need to let go of one day. We are all attached to something, most likely to lots of things, but the practice of *vairagya* tells us that we might want to rehearse letting go of our attachments little by little, as someday we will have to let go of every single thing we might think we are attached to.

Since joining the New England Sled Dog Club many years ago, I have rescued, trained, and raced retired sled dogs. I have always, for the past few years, named my white Siberian husky and main lead dog, Hopi, as the one thing that I am most attached to. I, of course, have always known that one day she would die. But as I practiced, training after training, year after year, with my students, letting go of my attachment to her, my dependency on her for joy, for happiness, for companionship, I began to love her and appreciate her more. But mostly, I began to find joy with her in the present moment.

Hopi died of lung cancer just before Thanksgiving in 2008. We found the cancer about a year before she died. After a major surgery in March, from which the vet and I thought there would be 100 percent recovery, two small metastatic tumors showed up on an X-ray in June. When I found out about the return of the cancer, I decided that I would walk with her every morning until the day she died. We would go out around 6 a.m. to the beach or the bay. We walked just to walk. Not to get anywhere, not as a means to an end, or for any purpose other than to be outside, with the sun and the wind and the seagulls and terns, and to be together. We did not put anything in front of us and run after it (except maybe a bunny or seagull) because everything we were looking for — peace, joy, love, happiness — could only be found inside us in the present moment.

The mornings were filled with brilliant sunshine or dark clouds. The waters were sometimes still and clear and sometimes turbulent and vague. We sniffed horseshoe crabs and seaweed. We peed on driftwood. Every moment was sacred, timeless. We sat together and watched the piping plovers fish for breakfast. We would smile and say hello to the pebbles, the blue sky, and the geese flying overhead. We would stop and breathe. We both knew that one day, the point of letting go that I had talked about for so long in my workshops, would soon come. But rather than sadness, that knowledge brought us to the present moment, (well not really "us" but me, Hopi always knew how to be in the present moment) and to an exquisite joy and fullness of life. Our hearts were mended and we were deeply at ease and happy.

I was in Florida in the middle of a week-long teacher training when I got the call from my dog sitter, Patrice, that Hopi wasn't doing so well. I changed my flight immediately and flew home, arriving just after midnight. Hopi did not greet me at the door, as she always did, and I prayed I would not go out to her kennel and find her dead. I walked out back and she came trotting around the corner, sooooooo happy to see me. Hopi and I had wonderful conversations all Thursday night, as I sat up with her until morning. We lit candles and built a fire in the fireplace.

She was having lots of difficulty breathing. She would not lie down and just stood outside, on the deck, and gazed into the distance, breathing with a shallow, but heavy rasping sound. I encouraged her to come in and lie down. With much persuasion, she would lie down next to me on her bed, and I would hold her head in my hand, stroking her ears and eyes gently. She would fall asleep — she was so tired and so fighting for life — and her breath would become silent and shallow. She would sleep, her head in my hand, for twenty or thirty minutes, then wake up, with her eyes big and a little frightened looking. She would stand and walk from one end of the living room to the other, then just stand, and struggle to breathe. I would encourage her, again, to come and lie down and, again, I would watch as she slept for thirty minutes or so.

I prayed her little heart would just stop and she wouldn't wake up. But she was an athlete, with a heart as strong as can be. She would wake again, then stand outside on the deck on that freezing cold night, and just try to breathe. I would let her stay out for ten minutes or so and then call her in. I was beside her as she tried to sleep five or six times. At 8:00 a.m., I called the vet and we planned for him to come to the house around 11:30. Then Hopi and I went for a walk — out to her training grounds — acres and acres of fields where we trained for our races every winter. Hopi ran lead on my team and was always the star of the show. She was an amazing lead dog and nothing distracted her. She had extraordinary focus when she was running.

She trotted around a bit — stopping and standing in the middle of the fields, with her head in the air, sniffing the wind - remembering all her training runs. She would trot a bit, and stop and rest. She came within fifty yards of a beautiful doe. In earlier days, Hopi would have been off like a rocket! This time, she and the doe just stood and regarded one another. We didn't stay long — about thirty minutes, then Hopi was ready to rest again. I told her it would be our last time together in these fields and that now she would go home and fall asleep and go on to her next adventures. I told her to choose her parents carefully and not to be born a starving or abused child — not to pick alcoholic parents or drug addicts or abusive parents — not to be born a suffering animal used for food or clothes or entertainment or medical studies to serve humans — to choose carefully — and find loving, joyful souls that would love her as I did, and as she did me.

The pain of her death was exquisite. I cried for weeks but felt an indescribable joy and comfort that was an equal part of the grief. I was so grateful that I had spent time with her — only with her, fully present and joyful.

I was grateful for my yoga practice in all its dimensions, for helping me to bear the loss of my best friend, and to embrace her death and understand it as a natural, normal, beautiful, really, part of life. I was able, thankfully, to celebrate impermanence as I cried.

ONLY ONE OF US HERE

Fundamental to quantum theory and one of the most significant parallels between the world of quantum physics and the ancient yoga teaching is in the idea of non-locality, or *connectedness*. Quantum interconnectedness is the idea that two quanta of energy, which are not in proximity (touching, or nearly touching), are connected. An experiment that proved this and has been repeated often demonstrates that two quanta of light, photons, given off from a single source and traveling at the speed of light in opposite directions, can maintain their connection to one another. What happens to one photon in the experiment, registers instantaneously with the other. I know that after my Hopi died, there was still a connection. Her spirit still touches me. It isn't my imagination. I have a deep knowing of the *connectedness* that transcends the physical world. I am sure many of you have experienced this same thing after the death of a loved one. I don't really need quantum physics to prove *non-locality* to me, as I am sure many of you don't either.

The quantum physicists are very careful to say that their research is confined to the world of quanta — things that are very, very small, and that these theories cannot be applied to the world of cosmology. Will science ever be able to prove that *connectedness* exists among us, among the planets, the galaxies, and even, yes, the universes? I don't know. I don't think so. I think the only way that that *connectedness* can be known is through the Inner Journey. And then once you make the discovery, see the "research" for yourself, how do you tell anyone about it? How do you prove it? You can't. I think it can only be proven to oneself, and the proof comes as a *knowing*, an awareness, which can't really be written down or formulated or calculated.

So how can we come to know *connectedness*? Quantum physics tells us that we are living in a non-local universe and yoga scripture tells us the same thing. But we want to have the *experience of non-locality*. Oh, sure, we can say that we know this, "Oh, I know all about non-locality, about the Gaia theory that says that the world is all One and connected to itself." And so you can adopt the worldview intellectually, and have it as a handy little bit of stimulating conversation that you trot out when you want to appear "spiritual." But unless you have experienced it, it doesn't really change you significantly, it just changes your worldview.

WHY ARE YOU DOING THIS?

Once we have worked through the early stages of yoga, which is essentially this physical practice of *asana*, a change begins to happen. If we have even made the smallest effort to pay attention, some tiny seed sprouts imperceptibly, and begins to grow. With continuing practice, a natural evolution occurs from gross to subtle, from the physical to the spiritual, from lesser awareness to greater awareness. Once this happens, we change. This change can take from six months to six years, but at some point, with regular practice, and there is absolutely no doubt about this, a process that I call "waking up" starts to unfold.

Since yoga is about paying attention and getting our attention into present time, there may be an instant when the mind becomes still. In that moment of stillness, there is a glimpse of a deeper reality, a peek of something beyond thought, when the attention comes to rest in the Now — a moment of recognition that we are organically connected to wholeness, a moment that goes beyond deliberations and worries over the past and future, a real glimpse of pure awareness that transcends time and space. If the experience is profound enough, there will be an actual spiritual *experience* of the true meaning of *yoga* itself, an experience of what is called, often in yoga, The True Self, or the revelation of perfect non-duality. Andrew Cohen, a well-respected spiritual teacher, defines the experience as, "that glimpse of ultimacy that awakens in us that recognition of our own true nature, One without a second." The light dawns, that's it.

Once we realize this connection, even for an instant, we become less self-centered and start to care about the world around us and the people in it. But although we may have experienced boundlessness for an instant, we understand that, although we have *experienced* the *state of* "yoga," we are still a long way from permanent residence in the *stage* of "yoga." This is the beginning of an arduous journey, but happily one that moves us from an egocentric, self-centered perspective to ever-increasing care and concern for greater and greater dimensions of life as a whole. Our circle of compassion begins to expand out into the world to include all sentient beings. That's the great thing. And we discover that that is what really makes us happy. Ultimately, it is serving others, doing for others, alleviating suffering — more than the biggest bank account or the biggest house or the utmost fame — that brings us the greatest happiness. That is why we do yoga. It is as simple as that.

THE CONVERGENCE OF ACTIVISM AND SPIRITUALITY

Traditionally spiritual seekers and social activists have walked different paths and at times even been disdainful of one another. If you were seeking God and the spiritual life, you were most likely going to follow a contemplative path and this meant "renouncing" the world and worldly pursuits. You went "off" to a monastery and sequestered yourself from the world and its temptations. If, on the other hand, you were an inspired social activist, you went out into the world to march for justice or equal rights or to save the whales or end the war or eradicate hunger or whatever cause you were fired up about. These two paths rarely intersected.

The truth is that we cannot possibly divorce ourselves from the world — we are the world! Today, if we are to any degree awake or spiritually conscious, we cannot avoid our responsibility of giving back to the rest of the world. There cannot be separation between these two paths. These two initially divergent paths are not divergent any longer. Already there is a mind-shift happening. I think to some degree we have the phenomena of yoga to thank for the shift that is occurring. I'm sure there are many other things to thank as well, but yoga and the way in which it works on a person's capacity for evolution, has definitely taken a primary role in the area of awakening people up to their global responsibilities.

Yoga is here now as a tangible methodology to wake us up. And once we wake up and realize that if one of us is hungry, we are all hungry, there is no going back. We can't go back and hang out in the bars, numb ourselves with drugs, or continue on any path that limits our ability to "be," to "know," or to be "blissful." We can't put our head in the sand so to speak. Well, we can of course, but it won't be quite as satisfying any longer. We have seen the light, and that picture haunts us, stays in our mind, calling us to higher levels of awareness. So our obligation, once we are awakened, is to *practice* — and that goes beyond the self serving aspect of simply evolving ourselves or liberating ourselves. We *practice* for the ultimate salvation of the human species. Now that might sound a little grandiose. But consider this:

The work of Rupert Sheldrake tells us that we are all connected through a morphogenetic field. The actions, thoughts, behaviors, and experiences of every species drop down into a "field" of energy that connects everyone within that species. It is similar to Jung's collective unconscious. We can all tap into that *field* — both consciously and unconsciously. Every time we *practice*, every time we make an effort to be mindful, we send *prana* down into that energetic aquifer. We add to the critical mass of that *field*. We are practicing for the Global Mind, not just ourselves. And every breath brings us closer to our own continuation, to the avoidance of extinction, and to the possibility of a quantum leap in Consciousness of the entire human species.

So we have an obligation to become *spiritual revolutionaries* — to awaken ourselves and then to go out and awaken the world, not through flag waving or proselytizing, but through right action, developed as a result of our *practice*. We have seen how what we discover about ourselves and the changes that occur during our *asana*, or *pranayama*, or meditation practice, are able to move out into the world with us and change our behavior in the world, not just on our mat.

In the ongoing teacher training program that is offered by my school, The Hard & The Soft Yoga Institute, part of every graduate's homework requirement, is to develop a Give Back project for their community, or a way in which they feel they can "give back" to their commu-

nity the benefits that they have been given by their teachers and their *practice* of yoga. These projects take all sorts of forms and are not by any means restricted to the teaching of *asana*. The projects range from people collecting surplus produce from the local supermarket that is about to be pitched, taking it home, cleaning it up through trimming and rinsing, and then taking it to homebound seniors; to distributing handcrafted, organic wool, yoga mat bags for a woman's cooperative in the rural mountains, just outside of Lima, Peru. Our Web sites, www.berylbenderbirch.com and www.boomer-yoga.com, list many of the Give Back projects that our students have developed and are working on. We also have links to other humanitarian organizations, animal rights organizations, or environmental organizations that we support or recommend. We also link to our nonprofit arm, The Give Back Yoga Foundation, www.givebackyoga.org which I started in 2007 with two of my students, Lori Klein and Rob Schware. Our objective is to provide funding for certified yoga teachers who wish to take yoga — in any form or practice — into the underserved or under-resourced areas of their community in some way, and need funds to do it.

A NEW ERA

On November 4, 2008, at 11:00 p.m. Eastern Standard Time, I was watching MSNBC, and NBC announced that Barack Obama had been elected president of the United States. It wasn't a jump-up-and-down-get-excited-moment for me; it was a deep contentment, a deep sense of gratitude and possibility. I started to cry. I stayed awake to watch Obama speak in Grant Park in Chicago. It was exhilarating and I think it was that way for most all Americans, even many of those who hadn't voted for the man. We, as a people, had decided, we had spoken, and it had worked. It was unbelievable.

To me it was a sign. I don't mean a big flashy sign like a chariot coming down from the skies with a big sign saying "Here is the message!" Just a sign. For years and years in my classes and workshops and trainings, I've been talking about the paradigm shift, the return to connectedness. I had felt like our collective practice, all of us together, was moving us towards the tipping point, the place where we reach critical mass and humankind will experience a quantum leap forward in Consciousness. Well, I don't know if everyone leapt, but it seems like about 52 percent of the population had a little jump that day. And then another little jump on January 20, 2009, the day of President Obama's inauguration. The joy, the connectedness filled almost every corner or the country. It was palpably historic. The energy of the planet was obvious. Friends called friends. People wanted to be with other people. Foreign countries were glued to CNN. There was a global interest in what was happening here in the U.S. The shift was happening!

Is it really possible that, along with science and spirit, on a socio-political level we might actually be moving towards greater awareness, through a bright, young, consciously evolved

politician with new ideas and compassion, who has captured the heart and hope of the country? I started thinking about the last eight years, and the moaning many have done about the mess that the narrow, fearful, and jingoistic governing style of the Bush administration landed us in. But I wondered. Maybe the past years will prove to be a good thing in the long run. Maybe the housing crisis, the economic crisis, and the Wall Street debacle forced us to wake up. It's almost like the Universe, tired of waiting for us to change voluntarily and become less greedy, less attached, more respectful, more compassionate — and more aware for heaven's sake — reached out with that ubiquitous 2x4 and bashed us over our collective global head. I think that the Earth was just plain sick and tired of being disregarded and desecrated. And now she is fighting back and we are coming face to face with our collective *karma* as a species. I think we are sick — both figuratively and literally, as individuals and as a culture — of being *disconnected*.

What has happened as a result? We are spending less and buying less gas. We've toned it down. Granted, we have been forced to, but it's happening. We're downsizing, we are growing food, we are looking to buy energy efficient cars, and we are becoming more aware of how each one of us is responsible for each other, our community, and the health of this planet.

The message from the Universe seems to be: spend less, quiet down, find contentment in simple things, and meditate more. To me it seems like it's all just starting to come together. Even in these grim times and with the large number of people who have lost their homes and their jobs and are so fearful about the future, there finally seems to be a light at the end of the tunnel. Does that mean we've seen the worst of the storm? I don't think so. Saddle up! It's going to be a rough ride and could get a lot worse. But what can we do? We are learning that a big house isn't who we are – it's comfortable, but we can get by with less. We are finding work in the new sectors of the economy. Sadly, industries like fishing for lobsters, building American SUVs, and logging for lumber may be close to over, but there is a ton of work to do. People are reinventing their lives. Unemployment is unimaginable if you think about all the work there is to do. It will just be different from what we are used to. How do we start?

Well, we have already started. We can get up in the morning, no matter what is going on, and instead of feeling fear or resentment, we can give thanks to God, or to our spirit guides, or our ancestors, or whatever we might feel the organizing principle of this Universe might be that gives us life, awareness, good health, and happiness. We can't always control the events of the world, but we can control what and where we put our energy and how we respond to the events around us. The work of yoga is to cultivate positive attitudes that may not be the first to arise in any given situation. Even if things are not going all that well, even if we are ill, or grieving, or depressed, if we can find the energy to be grateful for what we do have instead of focusing on what we don't have, we are well on our way to finding our own peace and happiness. That is the *spiritual revolution*. If we really work on cultivating gratitude, and replacing fear with a fullness of appreciation, it will move us towards greater clarity and wisdom. That's happiness. Am I *joyful*, you might ask yourself? Can I find joy today in spite of loss, or criticism, or pain? What is the choice? Who decides if not me? If we can do the work of a true *spiritual revolutionary*, and direct our attention to that part of us that is "awake" and "aware," then we can step out of our conditioned thoughts, and move towards happiness, freedom, and the *experience* of yoga. Aware presence, just now, just this! Hope to see you out there on the road! Safe travels.

Gate, gate, para gate
Para sam gate
Bodhe Svaha

(Beyond, beyond, go beyond
Go way beyond
Illuminate your Self)

— the last words of the Buddha

> "When the survival of the human race is in question, to continue with the status quo is to cooperate with insanity, to contribute to chaos. When darkness engulfs the spirit of the people, it is urgent for concerned people to awaken, to rise to revolution."
>
> — Vimala Thakar, *Spirituality and Social Action*

Index

Page numbers in *italic* indicate photos.

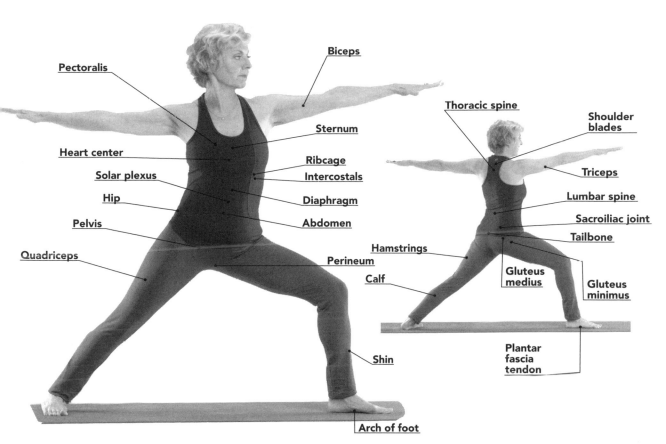

Anatomical Glossary

Abdomen: belly

Abduct: draw a limb outward

Adduct: draw a limb inward

Anterior: front

Arch of foot: inner side of the foot

Biceps: muscles at the front of the upper arm

Diaphragm: muscular partition that separates the chest area from the abdomen

Gluteus medius: one of the buttocks muscles

Gluteus minimus: one of the buttocks muscles

Hamstrings: muscles at the back of the thigh

Heart center: 4th *chakra*, center of the chest

Hyperextend: overextend

Intercostals: muscles between the ribs

Lumbar spine: lower back

Pectoralis: muscles that connect the front of the chest with the bones of the upper arms and shoulders

Pelvis; pelvic bowl: bony area near the base of the spine to which the legs are attached

Perineum: for men, the area between the anal sphincters and the scrotum; for women, between the anal sphincters and the vulva

Plantar fascia tendon: bottom of the foot

Posterior: back, backside

Psoas: muscle that runs from the lumbar spine through the groin and connects near the top of the inner thigh bone

Quadriceps ("quads"): muscles at the front of the thigh

Ribcage: bony frame formed by the ribs

Rotator cuff: muscles and tendons that connect the bone of the upper arm to the shoulder blade, includes the teres minor muscle

Sacroiliac: pair of joints located at the back of the pelvis

Shin: front of leg, below the knee

Shoulder blades: triangular bones positioned near the ribs in the upper back

Solar plexus: area at the base of the front ribs, above the belly

Sternum: chestplate

Tailbone: small bone at the base of the spinal column

Tendon: tissue that attaches muscle to bone

Thoracic spine: portion of spine roughly between the shoulders and the bottom of your rib cage (middle back)

Triceps: muscles at the back of the upper arm

Acknowledgments

As Mother Theresa once said, "You can do great things, but you can't do them alone." Community connects us all, creates gratitude, and gets us working together for the common good. Hopefully, that is what we have done with this book. Thanks so much to Sellers Publishing and to President and Publisher Ronnie Sellers for their confidence in and commitment to *Boomer Yoga*. From day one, Publishing Director Robin Haywood and the whole team at Sellers has been excited about and supportive of the project, and have worked hard to bring it to completion. Thanks to my brilliant editor, Editor-in-Chief of the Book Division, Mark Chimsky-Lustig. We worked together on *Power Yoga* and it has been wonderful to work with him again. Mark is the one who pulled all the elements together and drove the team home. And, of course, thanks to our production maestro Charlotte Smith and designer Heather Zschock, who turned text and photos into a beautiful book, and to Senior Editor Megan Hiller and Managing Editor Mary Baldwin for their heroic efforts. Thanks to our photographers François Gagné, Holly Haywood, and Bernie Meyers. Thanks to our stylist on our photo shoot, Lesley Tracy, and thanks to my walking buddy and student, Laura Berland, for the back cover author photo. Thanks to Michael Korda, Katie Couric, and Elizabeth Lesser for their support.

My tireless Executive Assistant Lori Klein needs baskets of thanks. She is a dedicated yogi, hard working and bright, and directs the organization and scheduling of my work. Thanks to my students (and graduates of my school) — our "models" Sheila and Tony Magalhaes, Jo Kirsch, Bob Speck, and Lori Klein (not a "boomer"!), and to all the 200- and 500-hour graduates from The Hard & The Soft Yoga Institute for their support. Thanks also to Corey De Rosa and his beautiful Tapovana Studio in Sag Harbor for a place to do "Mysore" practice in the mornings. Thanks to all my mentors and teachers, especially to Norman Allen, who, in 1980, taught me about the classical yoga practice of *astanga*. Thanks to my late husband Thom Birch, for adding music to my life and teaching me about focus, and thanks to all the people who host my workshops and trainings around the world. Special thanks to Dominator Clothing and Inner Waves Organics who sent us the many beautiful yoga clothes that you see us all wearing in the book. Thanks to my many dogs over the years, sweet Hopi, Nellie, Carmel, Cheat, Troy, Mo, Jesse, Gramfy, and Timber for the joy they bring and for showing me the value of the present moment. I am grateful to be able to work, and for the opportunity to travel and spread the teachings of yoga.